HPV and Head and Neck Cancer

Guest Editor

SARA I. PAI, MD, PhD

OTOLARYNGOLOGIC CLINICS OF NORTH AMERICA

www.oto.theclinics.com

August 2012 • Volume 45 • Number 4

SAUNDERS an imprint of ELSEVIER, Inc.

W.B. SAUNDERS COMPANY
A Division of Elsevier Inc.

1600 John F. Kennedy Boulevard ● Suite 1800 ● Philadelphia, Pennsylvania 19103-2899

http://www.theclinics.com

OTOLARYNGOLOGIC CLINICS OF NORTH AMERICA Volume 45, Number 4
August 2012 ISSN 0030-6665, ISBN-13: 978-1-4557-4924-9

Editor: Joanne Husovski
Development Editor: Donald Mumford

Otolaryngologic Clinics of North America (ISSN 0030-6665) is published bimonthly by Elsevier, Inc., 360 Park Avenue South, New York, NY 10010-1710. Months of issue are February, April, June, August, October, and December. Business and Editorial Offices: 1600 John F. Kennedy Blvd., Suite 1800, Philadelphia, PA 19103-2899. Customer Service Office: 6277 Sea Harbor Drive, Orlando, FL 32887-4800. Periodicals postage paid at New York, NY and additional mailing offices. Subscription prices is $335.00 per year (US individuals), $628.00 per year (US institutions), $161.00 per year (US student/resident), $442.00 per year (Canadian individuals), $789.00 per year (Canadian institutions), $496.00 per year (international individuals), $789.00 per year (international institutions), $248.00 per year (international & Canadian student/resident). Foreign air speed delivery is included in all *Clinics'* subscription prices. All prices are subject to change without notice. **POSTMASTER:** Send address changes to *Otolaryngologic Clinics of North America*, Elsevier Health Sciences Division, Subscription Customer Service, 3251 Riverport Lane, Maryland Heights, MO 63043. **Telephone: 1-800-654-2452 (U.S. and Canada); 314-447-8871 (outside U.S. and Canada). Fax: 314-447-8029. E-mail: journalscustomerservice-usa@elsevier.com (for print support); journalsonlinesupport-usa@elsevier.com (for online support).**

Reprints. For copies of 100 or more of articles in this publication, please contact the Commercial Reprints Department, Elsevier Inc., 360 Park Avenue South, New York, NY 10010-1710. Tel.: 212-633-3812; Fax: 212-462-1935; E-mail: reprints@elsevier.com.

Otolaryngologic Clinics of North America is also published in Spanish by McGraw-Hill Interamericana Editores S.A., P.O. Box 5-237, 06500 Mexico D.F., Mexico.

Otolaryngologic Clinics of North America is covered in *MEDLINE/PubMed (Index Medicus), Current Contents/Clinical Medicine, Excerpta Medica, BIOSIS, Science Citation Index,* and *ISI/BIOMED.*

Printed and bound by CPI Group (UK) Ltd, Croydon, CR0 4YY

Transferred to Digital Print 2012

Contributors

CONSULTING EDITOR

CHARLES W. CUMMINGS, MD
Otolaryngology–Head and Neck Surgery, Johns Hopkins School of Medicine,
Johns Hopkins International, Baltimore, Maryland

GUEST EDITOR

SARA I. PAI, MD, PhD, FACS
Associate Professor, Department of Otolaryngology-Head and Neck Surgery and
Oncology, Johns Hopkins University School of Medicine, Baltimore, Maryland

AUTHORS

SIMON R. BEST, MD
Assistant Professor, Department of Otolaryngology-Head and Neck Surgery, Johns
Hopkins School of Medicine, Baltimore, Maryland

CHRISTINE H. CHUNG, MD
Associate Professor, Department of Oncology, Johns Hopkins University School of
Medicine, Baltimore, Maryland

DIARMUID COUGHLAN, MPharm, MSc
Department of Health Policy & Management, Johns Hopkins School of Public Health,
Baltimore, Maryland; Department of Economics, National University of Ireland, Galway,
Galway, Ireland

GYPSYAMBER D'SOUZA, PhD, MPH, MS
Assistant Professor, Department of Epidemiology, Bloomberg School of Public Health,
Johns Hopkins University, Baltimore, Maryland

KEVIN D. FRICK, PhD
Department of Health Policy & Management, Johns Hopkins School of Public Health,
Baltimore, Maryland

DOROTHY GOLD, MSW, LCSW-C, OSW-C
Senior Oncology Social Worker, Milton J. Dance Jr, Head and Neck Center, Greater
Baltimore Medical Center, Baltimore, Maryland

ANDREW W. JOSEPH, MD, MPH
Resident Physician, Department of Otolaryngology–Head and Neck Surgery, Johns
Hopkins Medical Institutions, Baltimore, Maryland

WAYNE M. KOCH, MD
Professor, Department of Otolaryngology–Head and Neck Surgery, Johns Hopkins
University School of Medicine, Baltimore, Maryland

RYAN J. LI, MD
Resident, Department of Otolaryngology–Head and Neck Surgery, Johns Hopkins University, Baltimore, Maryland

KEVIN J. NIPARKO, AB
Dartmouth College, Hanover, New Hampshire

SARA I. PAI, MD, PhD, FACS
Associate Professor, Department of Otolaryngology-Head and Neck Surgery and Oncology, Johns Hopkins School of Medicine, Baltimore, Maryland

HARRY QUON, MD, MS
Departments of Radiation Oncology and Molecular Radiation Sciences, Otolaryngology–Head and Neck Surgery, and Oncology, Johns Hopkins University School of Medicine, Baltimore, Maryland

JEREMY D. RICHMON, MD
Assistant Professor, Director of Head and Neck Robotic Surgery, Department of Otolaryngology–Head and Neck Surgery, Johns Hopkins University, Baltimore, Maryland

DAVID L. SCHWARTZ, MD
Associate Professor, Departments of Radiation Medicine, Otolaryngology, and Molecular Medicine, Hofstra North Shore LIJ School of Medicine, New Hyde Park, New York

DONNA C. TIPPETT, MPH, MA, CCC-SLP
Assistant Professor, Department of Otolaryngology-Head and Neck Surgery; Department of Physical Medicine and Rehabilitation, Johns Hopkins University School of Medicine, Baltimore, Maryland

KIMBERLY T. WEBSTER, MA, MS, CCC-SLP
Assistant Professor, Department of Otolaryngology-Head and Neck Surgery, Johns Hopkins University School of Medicine, Baltimore, Maryland

WILLIAM H. WESTRA, MD
Departments of Pathology, Oncology, and Otolaryngology–Head and Neck Surgery, The Johns Hopkins Medical Institutions, Baltimore, Maryland

Contents

Human papillomavirus (HPV) is now recognized to cause a subset of head and neck squamous cell carcinomas (HNSCC). Although excessive tobacco and alcohol use continue to be important risk factors for HNSCC, epidemiologic studies suggest that more than 25% of HNSCC are now caused by HPV. The incidence of HPV-related HNSCC is increasing, highlighting the need to understand the oral HPV infections causing these cancers. This article reviews the evidence for a causal association between HPV and HNSCC, examines the changing epidemiologic trends of HNSCC, and discusses what is currently known about oral HPV infection, natural history, and transmission.

The confirmation of human papillomavirus (HPV) as a causative agent for a subset of squamous cell carcinomas of the head and neck has resulted in a growing expectation for HPV testing in head and neck cancers. An increasing understanding of HPV-related tumorigenesis has informed this evaluation process in a manner that is moving wide scale, indiscriminant, and nonstandardized testing toward a more directed, clinically relevant, and standardized approach. This review addresses the current state of HPV detection and focuses on the importance, appropriate time, and need for HPV testing.

Head and neck squamous cell carcinoma (HNSCC) that arises as a result of the activity of human papillomavirus (HPV) malignant transformation has a distinct disease pattern that is the basis for its clinical presentation. A clear understanding of these distinct clinical features enables diagnosticians to maintain awareness and index of suspicion to avoid delays in detection and select the most effective and thorough measures of evaluating the disease and directing treatment selection. Attention is focused on the broader demographic at risk for developing HPV-related HNSCC, the phenomenon of cystic cervical nodal metastases, and the unknown or occult primary cancer.

Patients with human papillomavirus (HPV)-positive squamous cell carcinoma of the oropharynx (SCCOP) enjoy better treatment outcomes than patients suffering from HPV-negative head and neck cancer. To maintain the integrity and utility of future clinical trials, HPV-positive SCCOP must be studied as a distinct entity. The discovery of HPV-positive disease has (1) convoluted comparison of current phase II trial data to historical controls, (2) made formal stratification for HPV infection status an imperative for future phase III trial design, and (3) drawn focus toward opportunities for personalization of treatment intensity. This review discusses these research issues.

This article outlines the biology of human papillomavirus (HPV) infection of human mucosa and the cellular pathways that are altered through viral infection. The article provides a conceptual framework with which to understand the 2 major immunologic strategies to address HPV-related diseases: (1) prevention of primary HPV infection through the use of prophylactic vaccines and (2) treatment of established infection and diseases through therapeutic vaccines. Nonimmunologic therapy that targets cellular dysregulation induced by HPV infection is also discussed. The challenges in actualizing these conceptually attractive therapies on both a societal and biological level are examined.

Surgery of oropharyngeal cancer has evolved from large, open transcervical and transmandibular approaches to minimally invasive transoral endoscopic techniques. Transoral laser microsurgery and transoral robotic surgery allow complete oncologic resection through the mouth with minimal cosmetic deformity and optimal speech and swallow function. With a significant increase in the incidence of oropharyngeal cancers, there is a growing role for up-front surgery, especially in young, healthy patients with human papillomavirus–associated squamous cell carcinoma. This article explores the development of transoral endoscopic surgery, its role in the multidisciplinary treatment of patients with oropharyngeal cancer, and oncologic and functional outcomes.

Past treatment efforts for head and neck squamous cell carcinomas have emphasized treatment intensification that increased local-regional control rates with an increased risk of late (swallowing) complications. With the improved survival demonstrated for human papillomavirus-related oropharyngeal carcinomas, strategies offering comparable outcomes but with fewer complications are needed. Radiotherapy dose reduction has been postulated to reduce the risk of late complications and is an active area of investigation. Alternative strategies may include the use of transoral surgery offering selective use of adjuvant therapy. This article summarizes the contributing risk factors of late swallowing complications and the strategies for risk reduction.

Swallowing and swallowing-related impairments present important post-treatment challenges in individuals undergoing organ preservation therapy for head and neck cancer. Literature pertinent to this topic is reviewed. A protocol for treatment of speech and swallowing deficits related to oropharyngeal cancer and treatment performed at Johns Hopkins Hospital is described. Data collected from a sample of oropharyngeal patients with cancer, with and without human papillomavirus-related disease, are summarized. Future directions for further study of this population are discussed.

Patients with head and neck cancer (HNC) suffer disproportionate psychosocial distress because of the nature of the tumor site, the possible impact on facial appearance and function, and the symptom burden resulting from treatment. Unmet psychosocial needs can negatively impact many aspects of care, from compliance to successful survivorship. This article reviews the challenges that patients with HNC confront throughout the disease trajectory from diagnosis to treatment, recovery, and long-term survivorship. It also provides a framework for understanding psychosocial adjustment and quality of life both for the general population of patients with HNC, and those with human papillomavirus-related diagnoses.

Cases of human papillomavirus (HPV)–associated head and neck cancers are rapidly increasing in the United States. Little is known about the economic burden of these cancers. A literature review identified 7 studies that characterized aspects of the overall economic burden of HPV-associated head and neck cancers in the United States. Other cost studies are detailed to highlight the clinical reality in treating these patients. As the clinical awareness of the role of HPV in head and neck cancers continues, the economic impact of cancers caused by this virus will have implications for the role of various preventive measures.

OTOLARYNGOLOGIC CLINICS
OF NORTH AMERICA

RELATED INTEREST

Impact of HPV status on treatment of squamous cell cancer of the oropharynx: What we know and what we need to know Silke Tribius, Anna S. Ihloff, Thorsten Rieckmann, Cordula Petersen, Markus Hoffmann. In: Cancer Letters, Volume 304, Issue 2, 28 May 2011, Pages 71–79

DOWNLOAD
Free App!

Review Articles
THE CLINICS

NOW AVAILABLE FOR YOUR iPhone and iPad

Foreword

HPV and Head and Neck Cancer

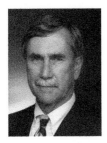

Charles W. Cummings, MD
Consulting Editor

I am extremely privileged to make a few comments about this particular issue of *Otolaryngologic Clinics of North America*. The topic of human papillomavirus (HPV) viral infection and its involvement with head and neck cancer has evolved from random concepts of inquisitive minds to a hard-edged, data-based association that encompasses modifications in the diagnostic process; fabrication of sophisticated schemes; and most importantly, confirmation of improved outcome statistics associated with HPV-related tumors of the head and neck. Dr Sara Pai and her coauthors have consolidated this evolutional process as it has matured at the Johns Hopkins Medical Institution. As a now senior and a molecular biologically out-of-touch head and neck clinician, I am awed by the progress that is being made in an area of oncology where I frequently hear that there has been no measurable improvement in outcomes and much less in the understanding of the basic tenets of head and neck cancers. The inextricable association of HPV viruses and a significant swath of oropharyngeal squamous cell carcinoma will most certainly affect concepts of prophylactic immunization globally over time. Welcome to this issue of the *Otolaryngologic Clinics*. You will be as pleased as I am with the contributions included here.

I am most sincerely,

Charles W. Cummings, MD
Otolaryngology–Head and Neck Surgery
Johns Hopkins School of Medicine
Johns Hopkins International
Baltimore, MD 21287, USA

E-mail address:
ccumming@jhmi.edu

Otolaryngol Clin N Am 45 (2012) ix
doi:10.1016/j.otc.2012.05.004
0030-6665/12/$ – see front matter © 2012 Elsevier Inc. All rights reserved.

Preface

HPV-Associated Head and Neck Cancers

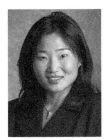

Sara I. Pai, MD, PhD
Guest Editor

The recent link between human papillomavirus (HPV) infection and a subset of head and neck cancers has ushered in new opportunities for the realization of personalized medicine. Advancements in the field continue to move at a rapid pace as the epidemiology of oral HPV infection and optimal detection methods for diagnosing the disease are better understood. Based on the distinct biology and pathogenesis of HPV-associated head and neck cancers, improved survival rates for patients with head and neck cancer are being observed for the first time in 40 years, and the field is transitioning into a new phase in which the focus is not only on achieving cure but also on improving the quality of life of these young head and neck cancer survivors. The importance of immune surveillance as a primary defense mechanism against cancer development is highlighted in HPV-related cancers. As increasing research efforts are made toward understanding the failed host immune responses against these virus-related cancers, strategies to reverse host immune tolerance and/or enhance immune recognition of these cancers can be evaluated. In the near future, HPV status undoubtedly will not only provide prognostic information but also guide treatment decisions, which will represent a tangible example of customizing health care based on the individual patient and the biology of his or her tumor.

The collection of authors contributing to this issue of *Otolaryngologic Clinics of North America* highlights the importance of multidisciplinary care in medicine and provides a detailed overview of state-of-the-art concepts in managing HPV-related head and neck cancer patients as practiced at The Johns Hopkins Hospital. We hope this volume helps to inspire open, educated communication among all practitioners who care for head and neck cancer patients, so that our shared goal of achieving the best possible care for patients is realized.

Otolaryngol Clin N Am 45 (2012) xi–xii
doi:10.1016/j.otc.2012.05.003
0030-6665/12/$ – see front matter © 2012 Elsevier Inc. All rights reserved.

oto.theclinics.com

This issue is dedicated to our patients, who have participated in and supported all of our research endeavors to deliver personalized medicine to the next generation.

Sara I. Pai, MD, PhD
Department of Otolaryngology-Head and Neck Surgery
Johns Hopkins University School of Medicine
601 North Caroline Street
Johns Hopkins Outpatient Center Room 6263
Baltimore, MD 21287, USA

E-mail address:
spai@jhmi.edu

Epidemiology of Human Papillomavirus-Related Head and Neck Cancer

Andrew W. Joseph, MD, MPH[a], Gypsyamber D'Souza, PhD, MPH, MS[b],*

KEYWORDS

- Human papillomavirus • HPV • Head and neck cancer • Oropharyngeal cancer
- Squamous cell carcinoma • Epidemiology

KEY POINTS

- In contrast to other head and neck cancers, the incidence of oropharyngeal malignancies has been increasing since the late 1970s, especially among younger men.
- The proportion of oropharyngeal cancers caused by human papillomavirus (HPV) is increasing; in many industrialized countries, up to 80% of oropharyngeal cancers are now caused by HPV.
- HPV-related head and neck squamous cell carcinomas (HNSCC) are more likely than HPV-unrelated HNSCC to occur in whites (93% vs 82%), never-drinker/never-smokers (16% vs 7%), those who have had more than 6 lifetime oral sexual partners (46% vs 20%), and those have a younger median age at cancer diagnosis (54 vs 60 years).
- The natural history of oral HPV infection is not well understood.

INTRODUCTION

Head and neck cancer (HNC) is a heterogeneous group of neoplasms that share a common anatomic origin. Although malignancies may arise from any tissue in the head and neck region, most tumors in this region develop from within the mucosa that lines the upper aerodigestive tract and are classified as squamous cell carcinomas. Head and neck squamous cell carcinomas (HNSCCs) include cancers in the oral cavity, oropharynx, nasopharynx, larynx, and hypopharynx.

Research over the past 15 years has shown that human papillomavirus (HPV) causes a subset of HNSCC, primarily oropharyngeal squamous cell carcinomas (OSCC). Although most HNSCCs are still caused by excessive tobacco and alcohol

Disclosure: G D'Souza has received research support from and is a consultant for Merck, Inc.
[a] Department of Otolaryngology–Head and Neck Surgery, Johns Hopkins Medical Institutions, JHOC 6th Floor, 601 North Caroline Street, Baltimore, MD 21287, USA; [b] Department of Epidemiology, Bloomberg School of Public Health, Johns Hopkins University, 615 North Wolfe Street, Room E6132, Baltimore, MD 21205, USA
* Corresponding author.
E-mail address: gdsouza@jhsph.edu

Otolaryngol Clin N Am 45 (2012) 739–764
doi:10.1016/j.otc.2012.04.003
0030-6665/12/$ – see front matter © 2012 Elsevier Inc. All rights reserved.

oto.theclinics.com

use, the incidence of HPV-related HNSCC (HPV-HNSCC) is increasing.[1,2] In some regions, HPV is now the primary cause of oropharyngeal cancer.[3,4]

In this article, we describe the changing epidemiology of HNSCC, examine the evidence supporting a causal association between HPV and HNSCC, and discuss what is currently known about oral HPV infection and natural history.

EPIDEMIOLOGY OF HNC
Overview of HNC Epidemiology

There are more than 600,000 incident cases of HNC worldwide each year, including ~263,020 oral cavity, 213,179 thyroid gland, 150,677 larynx, 136,622 pharynx, and 84,441 nasopharynx cases per year.[5] Nasopharyngeal cancers are often considered separately because of their distinct cause, related largely to infection with Epstein-Barr virus (EBV).[6] Thyroid cancers are also often distinguished from other HNCs because they are associated with separate risk factors and different causal pathways.[7]

The incidence of oral cavity, larynx, and pharynx cancer varies widely by geographic region and gender (**Fig. 1**).[8]

- HNC, ~90% of which are squamous cell carcinomas (HNSCC), has a 2-fold to 9-fold higher incidence among men than women.
- The age-standardized incidence of HNC is increased in South-Central Asia (14.1 per 100,000)[5,8] and in Melanesia (a region in the western Pacific Ocean, 22.1 per 100,000), because of high rates of tobacco use in these areas.[8,9]
- HNC incidence rates in the United States (9.9 per 100,000) and Europe (10.8 per 100,000) are lower than that observed in South-Central Asia and Melanesia, but remain notable.[5]
- Compared with the United States, HNC incidence is significantly lower in Micronesia (1.8 per 100,000), Middle Africa (3.4 per 100,000), and Eastern Asia (3.5 per 100,000), as well as throughout Western Africa (3.9 per 100,000) and Central America (4.7 per 100,000).[5]

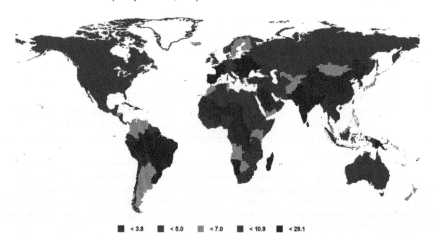

■ < 3.8   ■ < 5.0   ■ < 7.0   ■ < 10.9   ■ < 29.1

Fig. 1. World map from Globocan depicting age-standardized incidence rates (per 100,000 people) of cancers arising from the lip, oral cavity, and pharynx. (*Data from* Ferlay J, Shin HR, Bray F, et al. GLOBOCAN 2008 v1.2, Cancer Incidence and Mortality Worldwide: IARC Cancer-Base No. 10 [Internet]. Lyon, France: International Agency for Research on Cancer; 2010. Available at: http://globocan.iarc.fr. Accessed August 14, 2011.)

In the United States, an estimated 49,260 new cases of HNC were diagnosed in 2010.[10,11] Similar to worldwide differences in HNC by gender, the incidence of HNC in the United States is higher in men than women (15.9 vs 6.2 per 100,000). The median age at diagnosis of patients with HNC in the United States is in the seventh decade of life; however, the median age of onset is lower for cancers of the nasopharynx (55 years) and tonsil (57 years).[12]

Temporal Trends in HNC Incidence

Much of the geographic variability in HNC incidence may be explained by differential exposure to the major risk factors for HNC. Tobacco and alcohol exposure remain the most important risk factors for HNC overall, and are responsible for ~72% (95% confidence interval [CI]: 61%–79%) of HNC in the United States and Europe.[13] As a result of successful tobacco control programs, many industrialized countries have observed a decrease in per-capita cigarette consumption over the past several decades,[14] followed by a decrease in the overall incidence of HNC.[15] In the United States, cigarette consumption peaked in the 1960s; current tobacco use has been declining among both men and women, although use remains more prevalent among men.[16]

Following a decline in tobacco use, the incidence of cancer at many HNC sites has decreased in the United States. For example, between 1974 and 1999, there was a significant decrease in[17]:

- Lip cancer (from 2.7 to 1.1 cases per 100,000 people; $P<.05$)
- Oral cavity cancer (from 3.6 to 2.7 per 100,000 people, $P<.05$)
- Hypopharyngeal cancer (from 1.0 to 0.8 cases per 100,000 people; $P<.05$)
- Laryngeal cancer (from 5.4 to 4.5 cases per 100,000 people; $P<.05$).

In contrast to these decreases, the overall incidence remained stable over the same period for[17]:

- Nasopharyngeal: ~6 per 100,000 cancers
- Oropharyngeal: ~1.5 per 100,000 cancers.

In Europe, the incidence of oral cavity and oropharyngeal cancers has varied greatly by country and gender, with some countries experiencing increases in the age-standardized incidence rates over the last decade[18]:

- Males: England, Wales, Czech Republic
- Females: France, Netherlands, England, Wales, Denmark.

Other countries have observed decreasing incidences in rates over the last decade[18]:

- Males: Northern Ireland, Ireland, France, Finland, Norway, Slovenia, Spain
- Females: Malta.

Laryngeal cancer has been decreasing or remained stable in males and females from most European countries, with the exception of Swedish women, among whom it increased from 0.2 to 0.3 per 100,000 between 1994 and 2005.[18]

Changing Oral Cancer Incidence & Mortality in Selected Populations

Beginning in the 1980s, numerous reports from the United States and Europe began to document an increase in the incidence and mortality of tongue malignancies (both oral tongue and base of tongue) primarily among men younger than age 45 years.[19–22]

An increase in tongue carcinoma incidence has now been noted in multiple countries, including Scandinavian, Finnish, and US populations.[23-25] Furthermore, these increases are consistently shown to be most prominent among young (age 30–50 years) individuals. Among 30-year-old to 39-year-old men in the United States, the rate of mortality from tongue cancer increased 3-fold (0.3 vs 0.9, per 100,000 $P<.001$) between 1973 and 1984.[19]

Similarly, between 1973 and 2007, the incidence of oral tongue SCC increased in both male (annual percent change [APC] = +1.6, $P<.05$) and female (APC = +4; $P<.05$) patients younger than 44 years, although it was stable when not stratified by age and sex (APC = +0.1; P = not significant).[26] The increasing incidence of oral cancers has been observed among multiple countries, always in the younger age groups.[20,27-31] These increases are in stark contrast to the decreasing incidence of some other HNC subsites.

Tonsillar carcinoma incidence increasing

In the United States, data from the SEER (Surveillance, Epidemiology, and End Results) program showed that the incidence of tonsillar carcinomas increased significantly between 1973 and 1995 among both white (APC = +2.7) and black (APC = +1.9) men who were younger than age 60 years.[32] The incidence of tonsillar cancer among US women in the same period remained the same or decreased.[32] More recent analyses have reported similar increases. Between 1973 and 2001, the rate of tonsillar cancers increased significantly among 20-year-olds to 44-year-olds in the United States, from 0.18 to 0.25 per 100,000 (APC = +3.9; $P<.001$), whereas during the same period, the incidence at all other pharyngeal sites (excluding nasopharynx) remained constant or decreased.[25] Comparable increasing trends in oropharyngeal cancer have been observed in other populations, including studies from Canada, Denmark, the United Kingdom, Finland, Sweden, and Slovakia.[3,33-38]

Why is there an increasing incidence of oral cancers?

The increased incidence in oral tongue and oropharyngeal carcinoma is observed only for younger patients, with increasing rates noted especially among people born after 1950, although some studies have also suggested that people born between 1910 to 1950 have higher HNC rates than earlier generations.[19,20,28-32] Reasons for this cohort effect are not known. It has been suggested that changes in exposure to environmental carcinogens, such as smokeless tobacco products, might contribute to the increase in tongue cancers[19]; however, in the United States smokeless tobacco consumption has been declining among both adults and adolescents, so is unlikely to explain this pattern.[39] As discussed later, recent evidence suggests that an increasing proportion of these oropharyngeal cancers are caused by HPV. Changes in sexual behavior, leading to increased oral HPV infection, likely contribute to the increased incidence of oropharyngeal cancer.

ROLE OF HPV IN HNSCC
Evidence that HPV Causes a Subset of Oropharyngeal Cancers

Several different oncogenic HPV types have been identified in case series of HNSCC tumors[40]; however, greater than 90% of these HPV-HNSCC are associated with a single HPV type, HPV-16.[41] Estimates of the proportion of HNSCC that are caused by HPV have varied widely,[42] in part because of differences in case subsite composition, calendar year, country of study, and differences in tumor HPV detection methods. A systematic review of studies found that 26% of HNSCC have HPV DNA detected using polymerase chain reaction,[43] although this prevalence differs substantially by head and neck subsite.

Over the past decade, it has become clear that the increasing incidence of oropharyngeal cancers in developed nations is being driven by a new cause. There is clear molecular and epidemiologic evidence supporting a causal role for HPV in a subset of HNSCC. HPV is detected in the tumor cell nuclei, where it is transcriptionally active, clonal, and not found in the surrounding benign tissue.[44] In addition, case-control studies have shown that cases are more likely than matched controls to have current HPV DNA detected in their exfoliated oral cells, to have a higher number of lifetime oral sex partners (a surrogate for oral HPV exposure), and to have antibodies for HPV oncogenes.[45,46]

Studies have consistently shown that most HNSCC with HPV detected in tumor are from the oropharynx. The virus has an affinity for the lymphoepithelium of the Waldeyer ring, and in studies of HNSCC patients has been detected most frequently in oropharyngeal cancers. Most oropharyngeal cancers in the United States and Europe are now caused by HPV infection, although there is wide variation in the proportions reported by different US (36%–73%)[2,41,43–45,47–51] and European (14%–93%)[4,52–60] studies.

The proportion of oropharyngeal cancers caused by HPV seems to have increased over the past 30 years, suggesting HPV is driving the increasing incidence of oropharyngeal cancer recently observed.[4,61,62] A large Swedish study reported the prevalence of HPV detected in tonsil cancer increased from 23% in the 1970s, to 68% in 2000 ($P<.001$).[4] Additional increases of oropharyngeal cancers in Sweden being associated with HPV have been observed in the past 10 years[56]:

- 68%: 2000 to 2002
- 77%: 2003 to 2005
- 93%: 2006 to 2007.

Similar trends have been reported in several other studies,[61,62] including a study of US SEER tissues which showed that only 16% of US oropharyngeal cases had HPV detected in 1984 to 1989 compared with 73% during 2000 to 2004, a 4-fold increase in only 2 decades.[2] This study further suggested that the annual number of HPV-related oropharyngeal cancers in the United States is projected to surpass the number of incident invasive cervical cancer cases in the United States by 2020.[2]

Does HPV Cause Cancer at Nonoropharyngeal HNC Sites?

A causal role for HPV among oropharyngeal cancers is now established, but it is less clear whether HPV may cause HNSCC at other sites. Case-control studies evaluating the association of HPV DNA in oral exfoliated cells and odds of oral cavity or other non-oropharyngeal HNSCCs have most commonly been null[50,63–67] or small in magnitude,[65] unlike the strong associations observed for oropharyngeal cancers.[45,46,63,64,66,68–70] However, a role for HPV in a small subset of these cancers cannot be excluded because the etiologic heterogeneity of these nonoropharyngeal HNSCC sites would be more difficult to observe and some studies have suggested an association.[63] Initial studies have reported HPV detection in a subset of oral cavity, laryngeal, and nasopharyngeal cancers, but the consistency and strength of evidence implicating HPV at these sites are notably less than in the oropharynx.

HPV in laryngeal cancers

HPV DNA has been detected in 0% to 31% of laryngeal cancers in recent US studies,[44,71–83] whereas studies from populations in Europe, Asia, and elsewhere have reported higher prevalence estimates.[54,60,66,84–105,106–124,125–136] In addition to the data provided by these case series, a temporal relationship between HPV and the development of laryngeal cancer was suggested by 1 nested study of 76 laryngeal cases and 411 controls; this study showed that after adjusting for cotinine (a marker of nicotine exposure), individuals with serum HPV-16 antibodies were 2.4 times more likely than HPV-16– seronegative individuals to develop laryngeal cancer within 9 years from date of blood collection in the study.[66] Furthermore, a systematic review of the literature found that patients with laryngeal cancers were more likely than matched controls to have had exposure to HPV (odds ratio [OR] = 2.0; 95% CI 1.0, 4.2).[46] However, many of the individual studies had null results and they differed in their definition of exposure, for example[67,125,137–139]:

- Presence of HPV DNA in biopsy specimens
- Presence of HPV DNA in oral exfoliated cells
- Presence of serum antibodies against high-risk HPV.

Altogether, these studies suggest that HPV may be associated with laryngeal cancer, but it currently seems unlikely to cause a large proportion of cases in the general population. However, a special population of patients with recurrent respiratory papillomatosis (RRP) may be more susceptible to HPV-related oncogenesis in the larynx and other portions of the respiratory tract. RRP is typically associated with HPV types 6 and 11, which are considered to be low-risk types in the anogenital tract. However, data from clinical cases have documented instances in which low-risk HPV (typically HPV-11)-related RRP can undergo malignant transformation.[140–145] Nonetheless, even in this population, malignant transformation seems to be an uncommon outcome, with 3% to 5% of patients with adult-onset RRP and less than 1% of patients with juvenile-onset RRP developing carcinomas.[144–146]

HPV in oral cavity cancers

HPV DNA has been detected in ~25% of oral cavity cancers,[43,147] although the results of individual studies have varied greatly (**Fig. 2**). It is likely that these are overestimates, because some HPV-related oral cavity cancers show clear oropharyngeal involvement[148] and some of these oral cavity cancers are extensions from base-of-tongue primaries[15]; thus the proportion of oral cavity cancers that are HPV-related

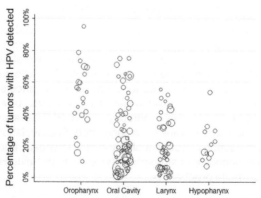

Fig. 2. Prevalence of HPV in tumors derived from the oropharynx,[2,4,44,45,47–60,197,198] oral cavity,[44,47,49,50,52,57,60,63,71,73,75–77,80,82,83,88,90–92,97,129,130,132,149,199–237] larynx,[44,71,72,74–76,80, 81,84,86,87,89–91,93–95,99–104,106,108,111,112,114–116,119,121,125,126,128,131,133,135,136,238] and hypopharynx.[54,75,76,80,83,85,97,100,107,108,132,239] Restricted to studies with greater than 25 subjects (oropharynx, oral cavity, larynx) or 15 subjects (hypopharynx) and which began enrollment after 1990. The size of each circle is proportional to the sample size of cases in that study.

is currently unknown. Several case-control studies have evaluated the association of HPV antibodies,[64,66-68,70,139] biopsy specimens,[149] or HPV DNA in oral epithelial cells.[63,64] The results of these studies have been varied, with some reporting a significant association between HPV and increased odds of oral cavity cancer,[63,64,66,70,149] whereas others studies found no significant association.[67,68,139] Therefore, it remains unclear whether HPV is a cause of a subset of oral cavity carcinomas.

For continuity with above formatting, we suggest you insert a subheading here with the following title "HPV in nasopharyngeal carcinomas." Recent studies have also begun to explore a potential role of HPV in nasopharyngeal carcinomas (NPCs). NPCs have classically been associated with EBV,[6] but HPV has also been detected in a subset (5%–83%) of NPC.[150-156] However, the few studies that have investigated HPV infections in normal nasopharyngeal epithelium have reported similar HPV estimates in benign nasopharyngeal tissues.[157-159] A recent study by Maxwell and colleagues[153] found that among 5 patients with NPC from a North American population, 4 harbored detectable HPV DNA and high p16 expression but lacked EBV-encoded RNA. These findings are consistent with a potential role for HPV in a subset of NPC from this population, but do not prove a causal relationship. In another recent investigation, Huang and colleagues[160] performed a case-control study and found no association between HPV and NPC in Taiwan. Therefore, there is insufficient evidence to support a causal association between HPV and NPC. Further studies are necessary to investigate this potentially important association. Nonetheless, given the potential for tonsillar carcinomas to extend into the nasopharynx, misclassification remains a challenge for these studies.

Role of HPV in the Changing Incidence of HNSCC

Given the strong role of HPV in oropharyngeal cancer and the small role of HPV in other HNSCC subsites, several studies have evaluated incidence trends after stratifying head and neck sites into those sites most likely to be HPV-related (subsites of the Waldeyer ring, including soft palate, palatine, and lingual tonsils) and those HNSCC sites where an HPV cause is unlikely (oral cavity, oral tongue). Chaturvedi and colleagues[1] found that between 1973 and 2004, the US incidence of HPV-HNSCC increased significantly (APC = +0.80, $P<.001$), especially among younger males (US incidence trends are depicted in **Fig. 3**). In contrast, the incidence of HPV-unrelated HNSCC decreased significantly during this same period (APC = −1.85, $P<.001$).[1]

In a similar study from 15 population-based European cancer registries, incidence trends of HPV-related HNC increased significantly between 1988 and 2002 (APC = +3.37, $P<.05$). HPV-unrelated HNC incidence in Europe also increased from 1988 until 1998 (APC = +1.73; 95% CI 1.2, 2.3), but seemed to plateau after 1998 (APC = −0.8; 95% CI −3.0, 1.5).[161] Studies using Canadian and Australian cancer registries also have observed increases in oropharyngeal cancer incidence.[34,162]

ORAL HPV INFECTION AND NATURAL HISTORY
Oral HPV Infection

There are more than 100 different types of HPV, distinguished by variations in their genetic sequence, and more than 15 HPV types that have been associated with human cancers.[163] HPV types are separated into high-risk oncogenic HPV types, including HPV-16, 18, 31, 33, 35, 39, 45, 51, 52, 56, 58, 59, 68, and 73; the remaining types are classified as low-risk or nononcogenic.[163,164] The carcinogenicity of HPV has been well described in the lower genital tract, where HPV is a necessary, but

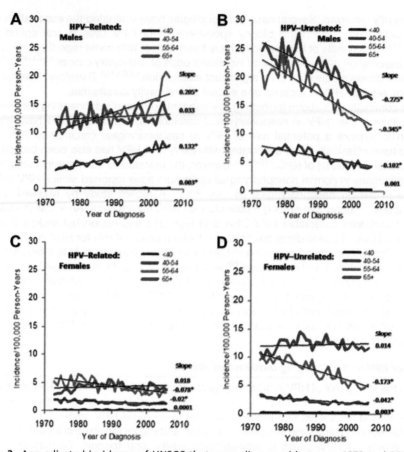

Fig. 3. Age-adjusted incidence of HNSCC that were diagnosed between 1973 and 2006 in males and females at HPV-related (*A*: males and *C*: females) and HPV-unrelated sites (*B*: males and *D*: females). HPV-related sites defined by International Classification of Disease for Oncology version 3 (ICD-3) codes for lingual tonsil, palatine tonsil, base of tongue, oropharynx, and Waldeyer ring. HPV-unrelated sites were defined by ICD-3 codes for unspecified and other sites of the oral cavity, including tongue, gum, floor of mouth, and palate. (*From* Marur S, D'Souza G, Westra WH, et al. HPV-associated head and neck cancer: a virus-related cancer epidemic. Lancet Oncol 2010;11(8):782; with permission.)

not sufficient, cause of invasive cervical cancer.[165] Although it is clear that HPV is an important cause of oropharyngeal cancer, infection with HPV is neither a necessary nor a sufficient cause of oropharyngeal cancer (oropharyngeal cancer can occur in the absence of HPV and not all oral HPV infections lead to malignant transformation).[166]

Several cross-sectional and case-control studies have sought to characterize the prevalence of oral HPV infections in the general population.[167–178] In a recent systematic review of 18 published studies, 4.5% (95% CI 3.9, 5.1) of 4070 healthy individuals had HPV DNA detected in oral exfoliated cells. The oral HPV prevalence was similar in men (4.6%) and women (4.4%).[179] High-risk oral HPV was detected in 3.5% of participants and oral HPV-16 infection was detected in 1.3% of all study individuals, representing approximately 28% of all oral HPV infections that were detected.[179] A recent large multinational study of healthy men reported slightly lower prevalence of[168]:

- Any high-risk oral HPV infection (1.3%; 95% CI 0.8%, 2.0%)
- HPV-16 (0.6%; 95% CI 0.2%, 1.1%) infection.

Higher oral HPV prevalence has been reported among select groups, such as:

- Individuals infected with the human immunodeficiency virus (HIV) (33%)[180]
- Current smokers (10%)[76]
- People with more than 5 lifetime sexual partners (7.4%).[76]

Natural History of Oral HPV Infection

Although the natural history of anogenital HPV infections and its transmission are well understood,[181,182] there have been few studies investigating the natural history of oral HPV infection. Initial studies suggest that some oral HPV infections may persist after more than 2 years, although the studies had limited power or did not include analysis by HPV type.[183,184] D'Souza and colleagues[180] investigated the 6-month natural history of oral HPV infections in a high-risk longitudinal cohort of 136 HIV-positive and 63 at-risk HIV-negative individuals. In this population, prevalent oral HPV infections detected at baseline were as likely as cervical infections to persist to 6 months among HIV-negative and HIV-positive individuals. Factors that were associated with increased oral HPV persistence included[180]:

- Current smoking status
- Older age
- Lower current CD4 cell count
- Use of highly active antiretroviral therapy (HAART) therapy
- Duration of HAART therapy.

These factors differed from those that predicted cervical HPV persistence at 6 months. For example, tobacco use was found to significantly increase the odds of oral HPV persistence, but not cervical persistence. Although this study population differs from the general population, it suggests that the oral HPV natural history or risk factors for persistence may differ in some ways from cervical HPV infection.

The long-term natural history of oral HPV infection has not been evaluated; however, initial studies suggest that, as with genital HPV infection, many infected people may clear their oral HPV infections quickly.[185,186] Further studies on oral HPV transmission, median time to clearance, and risk factors for persistence and progression are needed.

RISK FACTORS FOR HPV-HNSCC

Epidemiologic studies show that there are several notable differences in the demographics of patients who develop HPV-HNSCC compared with HPV-unrelated HNSCC patients (**Table 1**). Patients who have HPV-related cancers are on average[76,187]:

- Younger
- More likely to have a higher socioeconomic status
- More likely to have a higher education
- More likely to have more lifetime sexual partners
- Associated with white race.[187]

Table 1
Comparison of the general epidemiology of HPV-related and HPV-unrelated HNSCC

	HPV-HNSCC	HPV-Unrelated HNSCC
Incidence trend	Increasing	Decreasing/stable
Anatomic location	Primarily tonsil and base of tongue	All head and neck sites
Median age (y) at diagnosis	54	60
Socioeconomic status	Higher	Lower
Primary risk factors	Sexual exposure to oral HPV	Tobacco and alcohol exposure
Survival		
3-y oropharyngeal survival (%)	Better 82	Worse 57

Data from Refs.[1,34,45,76,161,162,187,188]

More specifically, the proportion of HNSCCs that are HPV-associated is significantly less in black compared with white patients (4% of black HNSCC vs 34% of white HNSCC in a recent study).[80]

Patients with HPV-HNSCC are:

- More likely to have an oropharyngeal primary tumor, to be diagnosed at a late stage, and to have better survival than those with HPV-unrelated HNSCC.[76,188]
- Less likely to have a history of extensive tobacco and alcohol use.[76]

However, despite these differences, most patients with HPV-HNSCC do have some tobacco or alcohol use; nonsmoker nondrinkers constitute less than 20% of patients with HPV-HNSCC.[189] HPV-HNSCC incidence rates are ~3-fold higher in men compared with women, similar to the 3-fold higher incidence of HPV-unrelated HNSCC in men compared with women.[1,190] Although increased male tobacco and alcohol use likely explains the higher incidence of HPV-unrelated HNSCC in men,[15] reasons for the higher incidence of HPV-HNSCC in men are less clear.

Given the different cause of HPV-related versus HPV-unrelated HNSCC, it is not surprising that the risk factors for these cancers are different as well. Increased sexual behavior (a surrogate for oral HPV exposure) has consistently been associated with increased odds of developing an HPV-HNSCC cancer.[45,50,65,167,175,191–193] Because sexual behaviors are colinear (people who have a higher number of partners for 1 sexual act tend to have a higher number of partners for other sexual acts as well), the associations with increased odds of HPV-HNSCC have been observed for various measures of sexual behavior, including:

- Earlier age of sexual debut[45,50,167,193]
- Higher number of lifetime vaginal sex partners[45,50,65,175,191–193]
- Higher number of lifetime oral sex partners.[45,65,167,175,191,192]

Given the colinearity of these behaviors, it is difficult to differentiate which sexual behaviors are associated with oral HPV transmission from these data. The strong association of sexual behavior with increased odds of HPV-HNSCC is not observed for HPV-unrelated HNSCC, which are primarily caused by alcohol and tobacco use.[76]

As HPV-HNSCC has become more common, the demographic profile of patients with HNSCC has begun to change from the traditionally older man who consumes tobacco and alcohol. Given the differences in patients with HPV-related and HPV-unrelated HNSCC, it might be tempting to assume that a younger, nonsmoking HNSCC patient is HPV-related or conversely that an older patient with a history of heavy tobacco use might be HPV-unrelated. However, a study exploring the predictive usefulness of age, race, tobacco use, and sexual history showed that these factors have only a moderate predictive value for true tumor HPV status. These factors had moderate predictive value among patients with oropharyngeal cancer (positive predictive value [PPV] = 55%, negative predictive value [NPV] = 68%) as well as when used among all patients with HNSCC (PPV = 75%, NPV = 65%).[194] Therefore, despite substantial differences in population characteristics, clinical HPV tumor testing is critical for determining whether the cause of the disease is related to HPV.

CURRENT CONTROVERSIES AND NUANCES TO HNSCC EPIDEMIOLOGY

There are several nuances and underappreciated aspects to the epidemiology of HPV-HNSCC.

Mischaracterization of Patients with HPV-HNSCC

Patients with HPV-HNSCC are sometimes mischaracterized by the press as highly sexual or promiscuous. Although the average number of sexual partners is larger among those with HPV-related versus HPV-unrelated HNSCC, the histories of individual patients vary greatly, and it is common for patients with HPV-related tumors to report a low number (<6) of lifetime sexual partners.[76] It is similarly important to note that only some patients with HPV-related tumors are nonsmokers/nondrinkers. Given evidence suggesting that smoking predicts higher risk of disease recurrence and distant metastasis in HPV-HNSCC,[195] counseling for smoking cessation should remain a priority for clinicians.

Race

Racial disparities in HNSCC incidence and survival remain striking. Because HPV-HNSCCs have been shown to have improved survival compared with HPV-unrelated carcinomas,[188] and a lower proportion of black patients diagnosed with HNSCC are HPV-related, racial differences in HNSCC survival may be in part or entirely explained by this difference in cause. Although initial studies support this possibility, suggesting survival of black and white patients with HPV-unrelated HNSCC is similar,[80,196] further investigation of these disparities is needed to understand whether there are differences in oral HPV acquisition or clearance.

Tumor Biology and Classification

There is some limited evidence to suggest that HPV may be associated with a small subset of HNSCC outside the oropharynx, although the results of these studies are far from clear. Furthermore, although HPV tumor status is clearly associated with improved survival among patients with oropharyngeal carcinomas, consensus around optimal biomarker profiles for HNSCC survival has not been established. Even more unclear is how to define patients with tumors who are HPV-negative but p16-positive. Because p16 overexpression is used by some institutions as a surrogate marker for HPV infection, are these tumors HPV-related despite the lack of detection of HPV DNA with the current assays? Further understanding of the biology of these tumors and how to classify them needs to be addressed.

FUTURE DIRECTIONS FOR EPIDEMIOLOGIC RESEARCH

In the last 20 years, a wealth of knowledge has emerged regarding HPV-HNSCC. HPV is now considered a cause of HNSCC, and the incidence of HPV-related oropharyngeal cancer is on the increase. Patients with HPV-related oropharyngeal carcinomas have better long-term survival, and may benefit from tailored therapies (reviewed elsewhere in this issue by Chung and Maurer and by Best and colleagues). However, our understanding of the natural history of oral HPV infections and their progression remains limited. In addition, reasons for the increasing incidence of HPV-HNSCC are not well understood. There is a clear need to institute better oral cancer screening techniques, which may help facilitate earlier detection.

SUMMARY

HPV-related carcinomas comprise at least 25% of all HNCs. Over the past 30 years, the incidence of oropharyngeal carcinomas has been increasing in many industrialized countries, and seems to be driven by an increase in HPV-related carcinomas. Oral HPV infections are sexually acquired and seem to be quickly cleared by most individuals but persist in a subset of infected individuals. The role of HPV in causing oropharyngeal cancer is clearly established, but it is less clear what role HPV may play in other head and neck subsites. Future studies that focus on the natural history of oral HPV infections could help to further our understanding of HPV-HNSCC. As tobacco-related HNSCC continues to decrease, HPV may continue to emerge as an increasingly important cause of HNSCC.

REFERENCES

1. Chaturvedi AK, Engels EA, Anderson WF, et al. Incidence trends for human papillomavirus-related and -unrelated oral squamous cell carcinomas in the United States. J Clin Oncol 2008;26(4):612–9.
2. Chaturvedi AK, Engels EA, Pfeiffer RM, et al. Human papillomavirus and rising oropharyngeal cancer incidence in the United States. J Clin Oncol 2011;29(32): 4294–301.
3. Hammarstedt L, Dahlstrand H, Lindquist D, et al. The incidence of tonsillar cancer in Sweden is increasing. Acta Otolaryngol 2007;127(9):988–92.
4. Hammarstedt L, Lindquist D, Dahlstrand H, et al. Human papillomavirus as a risk factor for the increase in incidence of tonsillar cancer. Int J Cancer 2006;119(11):2620–3.
5. Ferlay J, Shin HR, Bray F, et al. GLOBOCAN 2008, Cancer incidence and mortality worldwide: IARC Cancer Base No. 10 [Internet]. 2010. Available at: http://globocan.iarc.fr. Accessed August 14, 2011.
6. Young LS, Rickinson AB. Epstein-Barr virus: 40 years on. Nat Rev Cancer 2004; 4(10):757–68.
7. Schlumberger MJ. Papillary and follicular thyroid carcinoma. N Engl J Med 1998;338(5):297–306.
8. Jemal A, Bray F, Center MM, et al. Global cancer statistics. CA Cancer J Clin 2011;61(2):69–90.
9. Nair U, Bartsch H, Nair J. Alert for an epidemic of oral cancer due to use of the betel quid substitutes gutkha and pan masala: a review of agents and causative mechanisms. Mutagenesis 2004;19(4):251–62.
10. Jemal A, Siegel R, Xu J, et al. Cancer statistics, 2010. CA Cancer J Clin 2010; 60(5):277–300.

11. Fast Stats: An interactive tool for access to SEER cancer statistics. Available at: http://seer.cancer.gov/faststats. Accessed August 8, 2011.
12. Howlader N, Noone AM, Krapcho M, et al, editor. SEER Cancer Statistics Review, 1975-2008. Bethesda (MD): National Cancer Institute. Available at: http://seer.cancer.gov/csr/1975_2009_pops09/, based on November 2010 SEER data submission, posted to the SEER web site, 2011. Accessed April 19, 2012.
13. Hashibe M, Brennan P, Chuang SC, et al. Interaction between tobacco and alcohol use and the risk of head and neck cancer: pooled analysis in the International Head and Neck Cancer Epidemiology Consortium. Cancer Epidemiol Biomarkers Prev 2009;18(2):541-50.
14. IARC Working Group on the Evaluation of Carcinogenic Risks to Humans. Tobacco smoke and involuntary smoking. IARC Monogr Eval Carcinog Risks Hum 2004;83:1-1438.
15. Sturgis EM, Cinciripini PM. Trends in head and neck cancer incidence in relation to smoking prevalence: an emerging epidemic of human papillomavirus-associated cancers? Cancer 2007;110(7):1429-35.
16. NCI Monograph No. 8. Changes in cigarette-related disease risks and their implication for prevention and control. Report of the NCI Expert Committee. Bethesda (MD): U.S. Department of Health and Human Services, Public Health Service, National Institutes of Health; 1997.
17. Carvalho AL, Nishimoto IN, Califano JA, et al. Trends in incidence and prognosis for head and neck cancer in the United States: a site-specific analysis of the SEER database. Int J Cancer 2005;114(5):806-16.
18. Karim-Kos HE, de Vries E, Soerjomataram I, et al. Recent trends of cancer in Europe: a combined approach of incidence, survival and mortality for 17 cancer sites since the 1990s. Eur J Cancer 2008;44(10):1345-89.
19. Davis S, Severson RK. Increasing incidence of cancer of the tongue in the United States among young adults. Lancet 1987;2(8564):910-1.
20. Macfarlane GJ, Boyle P, Scully C. Oral cancer in Scotland: changing incidence and mortality. BMJ 1992;305(6862):1121-3.
21. Shemen LJ, Klotz J, Schottenfeld D, et al. Increase of tongue cancer in young men. JAMA 1984;252(14):1857.
22. Depue RH. Rising mortality from cancer of the tongue in young white males. N Engl J Med 1986;315(10):647.
23. Annertz K, Anderson H, Biorklund A, et al. Incidence and survival of squamous cell carcinoma of the tongue in Scandinavia, with special reference to young adults. Int J Cancer 2002;101(1):95-9.
24. Kari S, Alho OP, Jokinen K, et al. Carcinoma of the oral tongue in northern Finland: trends in overall incidence and patient and tumour characteristics. J Oral Pathol Med 1997;26(10):480-3.
25. Shiboski CH, Schmidt BL, Jordan RC. Tongue and tonsil carcinoma: increasing trends in the U.S. population ages 20-44 years. Cancer 2005; 103(9):1843-9.
26. Patel SC, Carpenter WR, Tyree S, et al. Increasing incidence of oral tongue squamous cell carcinoma in young white women, age 18 to 44 years. J Clin Oncol 2011;29(11):1488-94.
27. Franceschi S, Bidoli E, Herrero R, et al. Comparison of cancers of the oral cavity and pharynx worldwide: etiological clues. Oral Oncol 2000;36(1):106-15.
28. Hindle I, Downer MC, Speight PM. The epidemiology of oral cancer. Br J Oral Maxillofac Surg 1996;34(5):471-6.

29. Johnson NW, Warnakulasuriya KA. Epidemiology and aetiology of oral cancer in the United Kingdom. Community Dent Health 1993;10(Suppl 1): 13–29.

30. Macfarlane GJ, Boyle P, Evstifeeva TV, et al. Rising trends of oral cancer mortality among males worldwide: the return of an old public health problem. Cancer Causes Control 1994;5(3):259–65.

31. Mork J, Glattre E. Squamous cell carcinomas of the head and neck in Norway, 1953-92: an epidemiologic study of a low-risk population. Cancer Causes Control 1998;9(1):37–48.

32. Frisch M, Hjalgrim H, Jaeger AB, et al. Changing patterns of tonsillar squamous cell carcinoma in the United States. Cancer Causes Control 2000;11(6):489–95.

33. Syrjanen S. HPV infections and tonsillar carcinoma. J Clin Pathol 2004;57(5): 449–55.

34. Auluck A, Hislop G, Bajdik C, et al. Trends in oropharyngeal and oral cavity cancer incidence of human papillomavirus (HPV)-related and HPV-unrelated sites in a multicultural population: the British Columbia experience. Cancer 2010;116(11):2635–44.

35. Plesko I, Macfarlane GJ, Evstifeeva TV, et al. Oral and pharyngeal cancer incidence in Slovakia 1968-1989. Int J Control 1994;56(4):481–6.

36. Conway DI, Stockton DL, Warnakulasuriya KA, et al. Incidence of oral and oropharyngeal cancer in United Kingdom (1990-1999)–recent trends and regional variation. Oral Oncol 2006;42(6):586–92.

37. Robinson KL, Macfarlane GJ. Oropharyngeal cancer incidence and mortality in Scotland: are rates still increasing? Oral Oncol 2003;39(1):31–6.

38. Blomberg M, Nielsen A, Munk C, et al. Trends in head and neck cancer incidence in Denmark, 1978-2007: focus on human papillomavirus associated sites. Int J Cancer 2011;129(3):733–41.

39. Nelson DE, Mowery P, Tomar S, et al. Trends in smokeless tobacco use among adults and adolescents in the United States. Am J Public Health 2006;96(5):897–905.

40. Kojima A, Maeda H, Kurahashi N, et al. Human papillomaviruses in the normal oral cavity of children in Japan. Oral Oncol 2003;39(8):821–8.

41. Marur S, D'Souza G, Westra WH, et al. HPV-associated head and neck cancer: a virus-related cancer epidemic. Lancet Oncol 2010;11(8):781–9.

42. Syrjanen S. Human papillomaviruses in head and neck carcinomas. N Engl J Med 2007;356(19):1993–5.

43. Kreimer AR, Clifford GM, Boyle P, et al. Human papillomavirus types in head and neck squamous cell carcinomas worldwide: a systematic review. Cancer Epidemiol Biomarkers Prev 2005;14(2):467–75.

44. Gillison ML, Koch WM, Capone RB, et al. Evidence for a causal association between human papillomavirus and a subset of head and neck cancers. J Natl Cancer Inst 2000;92(9):709–20.

45. D'Souza G, Kreimer AR, Viscidi R, et al. Case-control study of human papillomavirus and oropharyngeal cancer. N Engl J Med 2007;356(19):1944–56.

46. Hobbs CG, Sterne JA, Bailey M, et al. Human papillomavirus and head and neck cancer: a systematic review and meta-analysis. Clin Otolaryngol 2006; 31(4):259–66.

47. Smith EM, Ritchie JM, Summersgill KF, et al. Age, sexual behavior and human papillomavirus infection in oral cavity and oropharyngeal cancers. Int J Cancer 2004;108(5):766–72.

48. Koch WM, Lango M, Sewell D, et al. Head and neck cancer in nonsmokers: a distinct clinical and molecular entity. Laryngoscope 1999;109(10):1544–51.

49. Ritchie JM, Smith EM, Summersgill KF, et al. Human papillomavirus infection as a prognostic factor in carcinomas of the oral cavity and oropharynx. Int J Cancer 2003;104(3):336–44.
50. Schwartz SM, Daling JR, Doody DR, et al. Oral cancer risk in relation to sexual history and evidence of human papillomavirus infection. J Natl Cancer Inst 1998;90(21):1626–36.
51. Strome SE, Savva A, Brissett AE, et al. Squamous cell carcinoma of the tonsils: a molecular analysis of HPV associations. Clin Cancer Res 2002;8(4):1093–100.
52. Cruz IB, Snijders PJ, Steenbergen RD, et al. Age-dependence of human papillomavirus DNA presence in oral squamous cell carcinomas. Eur J Cancer B Oral Oncol 1996;32B(1):55–62.
53. Fouret P, Monceaux G, Temam S, et al. Human papillomavirus in head and neck squamous cell carcinomas in nonsmokers. Arch Otolaryngol Head Neck Surg 1997;123(5):513–6.
54. Klussmann JP, Weissenborn SJ, Wieland U, et al. Prevalence, distribution, and viral load of human papillomavirus 16 DNA in tonsillar carcinomas. Cancer 2001; 92(11):2875–84.
55. Lindel K, Beer KT, Laissue J, et al. Human papillomavirus positive squamous cell carcinoma of the oropharynx: a radiosensitive subgroup of head and neck carcinoma. Cancer 2001;92(4):805–13.
56. Nasman A, Attner P, Hammarstedt L, et al. Incidence of human papillomavirus (HPV) positive tonsillar carcinoma in Stockholm, Sweden: an epidemic of viral-induced carcinoma? Int J Cancer 2009;125(2):362–6.
57. Romanitan M, Nasman A, Ramqvist T, et al. Human papillomavirus frequency in oral and oropharyngeal cancer in Greece. Anticancer Res 2008;28(4B): 2077–80.
58. Tachezy R, Klozar J, Rubenstein L, et al. Demographic and risk factors in patients with head and neck tumors. J Med Virol 2009;81(5):878–87.
59. Tachezy R, Klozar J, Salakova M, et al. HPV and other risk factors of oral cavity/oropharyngeal cancer in the Czech Republic. Oral Dis 2005;11(3):181–5.
60. van Houten VM, Snijders PJ, van den Brekel MW, et al. Biological evidence that human papillomaviruses are etiologically involved in a subgroup of head and neck squamous cell carcinomas. Int J Cancer 2001;93(2):232–5.
61. Ernster JA, Sciotto CG, O'Brien MM, et al. Rising incidence of oropharyngeal cancer and the role of oncogenic human papilloma virus. Laryngoscope 2007;117(12):2115–28.
62. Lundberg M, Leivo I, Saarilahti K, et al. Increased incidence of oropharyngeal cancer and p16 expression. Acta Otolaryngol 2011;131(9):1008–11.
63. Hansson BG, Rosenquist K, Antonsson A, et al. Strong association between infection with human papillomavirus and oral and oropharyngeal squamous cell carcinoma: a population-based case-control study in southern Sweden. Acta Otolaryngol 2005;125(12):1337–44.
64. Herrero R, Castellsague X, Pawlita M, et al. Human papillomavirus and oral cancer: the International Agency for Research on Cancer multicenter study. J Natl Cancer Inst 2003;95(23):1772–83.
65. Maden C, Beckmann AM, Thomas DB, et al. Human papillomaviruses, herpes simplex viruses, and the risk of oral cancer in men. Am J Epidemiol 1992; 135(10):1093–102.
66. Mork J, Lie AK, Glattre E, et al. Human papillomavirus infection as a risk factor for squamous-cell carcinoma of the head and neck. N Engl J Med 2001;344(15): 1125–31.

67. Van Doornum GJ, Korse CM, Buning-Kager JC, et al. Reactivity to human papillomavirus type 16 L1 virus-like particles in sera from patients with genital cancer and patients with carcinomas at five different extragenital sites. Br J Cancer 2003;88(7):1095–100.

68. Dahlstrom KR, Adler-Storthz K, Etzel CJ, et al. Human papillomavirus type 16 infection and squamous cell carcinoma of the head and neck in never-smokers: a matched pair analysis. Clin Cancer Res 2003;9(7):2620–6.

69. Smith EM, Ritchie JM, Summersgill KF, et al. Human papillomavirus in oral exfoliated cells and risk of head and neck cancer. J Natl Cancer Inst 2004;96(6):449–55.

70. Smith EM, Ritchie JM, Pawlita M, et al. Human papillomavirus seropositivity and risks of head and neck cancer. Int J Cancer 2007;120(4):825–32.

71. Agrawal Y, Koch WM, Xiao W, et al. Oral human papillomavirus infection before and after treatment for human papillomavirus 16-positive and human papillomavirus 16-negative head and neck squamous cell carcinoma. Clin Cancer Res 2008;14(21):7143–50.

72. Baumann JL, Cohen S, Evjen AN, et al. Human papillomavirus in early laryngeal carcinoma. Laryngoscope 2009;119(8):1531–7.

73. Capone RB, Pai SI, Koch WM, et al. Detection and quantitation of human papillomavirus (HPV) DNA in the sera of patients with HPV-associated head and neck squamous cell carcinoma. Clin Cancer Res 2000;6(11):4171–5.

74. Fakhry C, Westra WH, Li S, et al. Improved survival of patients with human papillomavirus-positive head and neck squamous cell carcinoma in a prospective clinical trial. J Natl Cancer Inst 2008;100(4):261–9.

75. Furniss CS, McClean MD, Smith JF, et al. Human papillomavirus 16 and head and neck squamous cell carcinoma. Int J Cancer 2007;120(11):2386–92.

76. Gillison ML, D'Souza G, Westra W, et al. Distinct risk factor profiles for human papillomavirus type 16-positive and human papillomavirus type 16-negative head and neck cancers. J Natl Cancer Inst 2008;100(6):407–20.

77. Haraf DJ, Nodzenski E, Brachman D, et al. Human papilloma virus and p53 in head and neck cancer: clinical correlates and survival. Clin Cancer Res 1996;2(4):755–62.

78. Olshan AF, Weissler MC, Pei H, et al. Alterations of the p16 gene in head and neck cancer: frequency and association with p53, PRAD-1 and HPV. Oncogene 1997;14(7):811–8.

79. Paz IB, Cook N, Odom-Maryon T, et al. Human papillomavirus (HPV) in head and neck cancer. An association of HPV 16 with squamous cell carcinoma of Waldeyer's tonsillar ring. Cancer 1997;79(3):595–604.

80. Settle K, Posner MR, Schumaker LM, et al. Racial survival disparity in head and neck cancer results from low prevalence of human papillomavirus infection in black oropharyngeal cancer patients. Cancer Prev Res (Phila) 2009;2(9):776–81.

81. Shen J, Tate JE, Crum CP, et al. Prevalence of human papillomaviruses (HPV) in benign and malignant tumors of the upper respiratory tract. Mod Pathol 1996;9(1):15–20.

82. Westra WH, Taube JM, Poeta ML, et al. Inverse relationship between human papillomavirus-16 infection and disruptive p53 gene mutations in squamous cell carcinoma of the head and neck. Clin Cancer Res 2008;14(2):366–9.

83. Zhao M, Rosenbaum E, Carvalho AL, et al. Feasibility of quantitative PCR-based saliva rinse screening of HPV for head and neck cancer. Int J Cancer 2005;117(4):605–10.

84. Almadori G, Cadoni G, Cattani P, et al. Detection of human papillomavirus DNA in laryngeal squamous cell carcinoma by polymerase chain reaction. Eur J Cancer 1996;32A(5):783–8.

85. Alvarez Alvarez I, Sanchez Lazo P, Ramos Gonzalez S, et al. Using polymerase chain reaction to human papillomavirus in oral and pharyngolaryngeal carcinomas. Am J Otolaryngol 1997;18(6):375–81.

86. Anderson CE, McLaren KM, Rae F, et al. Human papilloma virus in squamous carcinoma of the head and neck: a study of cases in south east Scotland. J Clin Pathol 2007;60(4):439–41.

87. Anwar K, Nakakuki K, Naiki H, et al. ras gene mutations and HPV infection are common in human laryngeal carcinoma. Int J Cancer 1993;53(1):22–8.

88. Atula S, Auvinen E, Grenman R, et al. Human papillomavirus and Epstein-Barr virus in epithelial carcinomas of the head and neck region. Anticancer Res 1997;17(6D):4427–33.

89. Azzimonti B, Pagano M, Mondini M, et al. Altered patterns of the interferon-inducible gene IFI16 expression in head and neck squamous cell carcinoma: immunohistochemical study including correlation with retinoblastoma protein, human papillomavirus infection and proliferation index. Histopathology 2004; 45(6):560–72.

90. Badaracco G, Rizzo C, Mafera B, et al. Molecular analyses and prognostic relevance of HPV in head and neck tumours. Oncol Rep 2007;17(4):931–9.

91. Baez A, Almodovar JI, Cantor A, et al. High frequency of HPV16-associated head and neck squamous cell carcinoma in the Puerto Rican population. Head Neck 2004;26(9):778–84.

92. Bhattacharya N, Roy A, Roy B, et al. MYC gene amplification reveals clinical association with head and neck squamous cell carcinoma in Indian patients. J Oral Pathol Med 2009;38(10):759–63.

93. Boscolo-Rizzo P, Da Mosto MC, Fuson R, et al. HPV-16 E6 L83V variant in squamous cell carcinomas of the upper aerodigestive tract. J Cancer Res Clin Oncol 2009;135(4):559–66.

94. Cattani P, Hohaus S, Bellacosa A, et al. Association between cyclin D1 (CCND1) gene amplification and human papillomavirus infection in human laryngeal squamous cell carcinoma. Clin Cancer Res 1998;4(11):2585–9.

95. Cerovac Z, Sarcevic B, Kralj Z, et al. Detection of human papillomavirus (HPV) type 6, 16 and 18 in head and neck squamous cell carcinomas by in situ hybridization. Neoplasma 1996;43(3):185–94.

96. de Oliveira DE, Bacchi MM, Macarenco RS, et al. Human papillomavirus and Epstein-Barr virus infection, p53 expression, and cellular proliferation in laryngeal carcinoma. Am J Clin Pathol 2006;126(2):284–93.

97. Deng Z, Hasegawa M, Matayoshi S, et al. Prevalence and clinical features of human papillomavirus in head and neck squamous cell carcinoma in Okinawa, southern Japan. Eur Arch Otorhinolaryngol 2011;268(11):1625–31.

98. Fischer M. Analysis of exon 2 of MTS1 in HPV-positive and HPV-negative tumors of the head and neck region. Eur Arch Otorhinolaryngol 2007;264(7):801–7.

99. Fischer M, von Winterfeld F. Evaluation and application of a broad-spectrum polymerase chain reaction assay for human papillomaviruses in the screening of squamous cell tumours of the head and neck. Acta Otolaryngol 2003; 123(6):752–8.

100. Fouret P, Martin F, Flahault A, et al. Human papillomavirus infection in the malignant and premalignant head and neck epithelium. Diagn Mol Pathol 1995;4(2): 122–7.

101. Gallo A, Degener AM, Pagliuca G, et al. Detection of human papillomavirus and adenovirus in benign and malignant lesions of the larynx. Otolaryngol Head Neck Surg 2009;141(2):276–81.

102. Garcia-Milian R, Hernandez H, Panade L, et al. Detection and typing of human papillomavirus DNA in benign and malignant tumours of laryngeal epithelium. Acta Otolaryngol 1998;118(5):754–8.

103. Gorgoulis V, Rassidakis G, Karameris A, et al. Expression of p53 protein in laryngeal squamous cell carcinoma and dysplasia: possible correlation with human papillomavirus infection and clinicopathological findings. Virchows Arch 1994; 425(5):481–9.

104. Gorgoulis VG, Zacharatos P, Kotsinas A, et al. Human papilloma virus (HPV) is possibly involved in laryngeal but not in lung carcinogenesis. Hum Pathol 1999; 30(3):274–83.

105. Gudleviciene Z, Smailyte G, Mickonas A, et al. Prevalence of human papillomavirus and other risk factors in Lithuanian patients with head and neck cancer. Oncology 2009;76(3):205–8.

106. Guvenc MG, Midilli K, Ozdogan A, et al. Detection of HHV-8 and HPV in laryngeal carcinoma. Auris Nasus Larynx 2008;35(3):357–62.

107. Hoffmann M, Gorogh T, Gottschlich S, et al. Human papillomaviruses in head and neck cancer: 8 year-survival-analysis of 73 patients. Cancer Lett 2005; 218(2):199–206.

108. Hoffmann M, Kahn T, Mahnke CG, et al. Prevalence of human papillomavirus in squamous cell carcinoma of the head and neck determined by polymerase chain reaction and Southern blot hybridization: proposal for optimized diagnostic requirements. Acta Otolaryngol 1998;118(1):138–44.

109. Hoffmann M, Orlamunder A, Sucher J, et al. HPV16 DNA in histologically confirmed tumour-free neck lymph nodes of head and neck cancers. Anticancer Res 2006;26(1B):663–70.

110. Hoffmann M, Scheunemann D, Fazel A, et al. Human papillomavirus and p53 polymorphism in codon 72 in head and neck squamous cell carcinoma. Oncol Rep 2009;21(3):809–14.

111. Kleist B, Poetsch M, Bankau A, et al. First hints for a correlation between amplification of the Int-2 gene and infection with human papillomavirus in head and neck squamous cell carcinomas. J Oral Pathol Med 2000;29(9): 432–7.

112. Koskinen WJ, Brondbo K, Mellin Dahlstrand H, et al. Alcohol, smoking and human papillomavirus in laryngeal carcinoma: a Nordic prospective multicenter study. J Cancer Res Clin Oncol 2007;133(9):673–8.

113. Koskinen WJ, Chen RW, Leivo I, et al. Prevalence and physical status of human papillomavirus in squamous cell carcinomas of the head and neck. Int J Cancer 2003;107(3):401–6.

114. Lee SY, Cho NH, Choi EC, et al. Is human papillomavirus a causative factor of glottic cancer? J Voice 2011;25(6):770–4.

115. Lie ES, Karlsen F, Holm R. Presence of human papillomavirus in squamous cell laryngeal carcinomas. A study of thirty-nine cases using polymerase chain reaction and in situ hybridization. Acta Otolaryngol 1996;116(6):900–5.

116. Lindeberg H, Krogdahl A. Laryngeal cancer and human papillomavirus: HPV is absent in the majority of laryngeal carcinomas. Cancer Lett 1999;146(1): 9–13.

117. Major T, Szarka K, Sziklai I, et al. The characteristics of human papillomavirus DNA in head and neck cancers and papillomas. J Clin Pathol 2005;58(1):51–5.

118. Manjarrez ME, Ocadiz R, Valle L, et al. Detection of human papillomavirus and relevant tumor suppressors and oncoproteins in laryngeal tumors. Clin Cancer Res 2006;12(23):6946–51.

119. Miranda FA, Hassumi MK, Guimaraes MC, et al. Galectin-3 overexpression in invasive laryngeal carcinoma, assessed by computer-assisted analysis. J Histochem Cytochem 2009;57(7):665–73.

120. Mitra S, Banerjee S, Misra C, et al. Interplay between human papilloma virus infection and p53 gene alterations in head and neck squamous cell carcinoma of an Indian patient population. J Clin Pathol 2007;60(9):1040–7.

121. Morshed K. Association between human papillomavirus infection and laryngeal squamous cell carcinoma. J Med Virol 2010;82(6):1017–23.

122. Morshed K, Korobowicz E, Szymanski M, et al. Immunohistochemical demonstration of multiple HPV types in laryngeal squamous cell carcinoma. Eur Arch Otorhinolaryngol 2005;262(11):917–20.

123. Morshed K, Polz-Dacewicz M, Szymanski M, et al. Short-fragment PCR assay for highly sensitive broad-spectrum detection of human papillomaviruses in laryngeal squamous cell carcinoma and normal mucosa: clinico-pathological evaluation. Eur Arch Otorhinolaryngol 2008;265(Suppl 1):S89–96.

124. Morshed K, Polz-Dacewicz M, Szymanski M, et al. Usefulness and efficiency of formalin-fixed paraffin-embedded specimens from laryngeal squamous cell carcinoma in HPV detection by IHC and PCR/DEIA. Folia Histochem Cytobiol 2010;48(3):398–402.

125. Nishioka S, Fukushima K, Nishizaki K, et al. Human papillomavirus as a risk factor for head and neck cancers–a case-control study. Acta Otolaryngol Suppl 1999;540:77–80.

126. Ogura H, Watanabe S, Fukushima K, et al. Presence of human papillomavirus type 18 DNA in a pharyngeal and a laryngeal carcinoma. Jpn J Cancer Res 1991;82(11):1184–6.

127. Peralta R, Baudis M, Vazquez G, et al. Increased expression of cellular retinol-binding protein 1 in laryngeal squamous cell carcinoma. J Cancer Res Clin Oncol 2010;136(6):931–8.

128. Poljak M, Gale N, Kambic V. Human papillomaviruses: a study of their prevalence in the epithelial hyperplastic lesions of the larynx. Acta Otolaryngol Suppl 1997;527:66–9.

129. Ritta M, De Andrea M, Mondini M, et al. Cell cycle and viral and immunologic profiles of head and neck squamous cell carcinoma as predictable variables of tumor progression. Head Neck 2009;31(3):318–27.

130. Sabbir MG, Dasgupta S, Roy A, et al. Genetic alterations (amplification and rearrangement) of D-type cyclins loci in head and neck squamous cell carcinoma of Indian patients: prognostic significance and clinical implications. Diagn Mol Pathol 2006;15(1):7–16.

131. Salam MA, Rockett J, Morris A. General primer-mediated polymerase chain reaction for simultaneous detection and typing of human papillomavirus DNA in laryngeal squamous cell carcinomas. Clin Otolaryngol Allied Sci 1995; 20(1):84–8.

132. Snijders PJ, Scholes AG, Hart CA, et al. Prevalence of mucosotropic human papillomaviruses in squamous-cell carcinoma of the head and neck. Int J Cancer 1996;66(4):464–9.

133. Torrente MC, Ampuero S, Abud M, et al. Molecular detection and typing of human papillomavirus in laryngeal carcinoma specimens. Acta Otolaryngol 2005;125(8):888–93.

134. Tyan YS, Liu ST, Ong WR, et al. Detection of Epstein-Barr virus and human papillomavirus in head and neck tumors. J Clin Microbiol 1993;31(1):53–6.

135. Venuti A, Manni V, Morello R, et al. Physical state and expression of human papillomavirus in laryngeal carcinoma and surrounding normal mucosa. J Med Virol 2000;60(4):396–402.

136. Vlachtsis K, Nikolaou A, Markou K, et al. Clinical and molecular prognostic factors in operable laryngeal cancer. Eur Arch Otorhinolaryngol 2005;262(11):890–8.

137. Brandsma JL, Abramson AL. Association of papillomavirus with cancers of the head and neck. Arch Otolaryngol Head Neck Surg 1989;115(5):621–5.

138. Smith EM, Summersgill KF, Allen J, et al. Human papillomavirus and risk of laryngeal cancer. Ann Otol Rhinol Laryngol 2000;109(11):1069–76.

139. Dillner J, Knekt P, Schiller JT, et al. Prospective seroepidemiological evidence that human papillomavirus type 16 infection is a risk factor for oesophageal squamous cell carcinoma. BMJ 1995;311(7016):1346.

140. Cook JR, Hill DA, Humphrey PA, et al. Squamous cell carcinoma arising in recurrent respiratory papillomatosis with pulmonary involvement: emerging common pattern of clinical features and human papillomavirus serotype association. Mod Pathol 2000;13(8):914–8.

141. Lin HW, Richmon JD, Emerick KS, et al. Malignant transformation of a highly aggressive human papillomavirus type 11-associated recurrent respiratory papillomatosis. Am J Otolaryngol 2010;31(4):291–6.

142. Reidy PM, Dedo HH, Rabah R, et al. Integration of human papillomavirus type 11 in recurrent respiratory papilloma-associated cancer. Laryngoscope 2004; 114(11):1906–9.

143. Gerein V, Rastorguev E, Gerein J, et al. Use of interferon-alpha in recurrent respiratory papillomatosis: 20-year follow-up. Ann Otol Rhinol Laryngol 2005; 114(6):463–71.

144. Klozar J, Taudy M, Betka J, et al. Laryngeal papilloma–precancerous condition? Acta Otolaryngol Suppl 1997;527:100–2.

145. Hartley C, Hamilton J, Birzgalis AR, et al. Recurrent respiratory papillomatosis–the Manchester experience, 1974-1992. J Laryngol Otol 1994;108(3):226–9.

146. Donne AJ, Hampson L, Homer JJ, et al. The role of HPV type in Recurrent Respiratory Papillomatosis. Int J Pediatr Otorhinolaryngol 2010;74(1):7–14.

147. Torrente MC, Rodrigo JP, Haigentz M Jr, et al. Human papillomavirus infections in laryngeal cancer. Head Neck 2011;33(4):581–6.

148. Lopes V, Murray P, Williams H, et al. Squamous cell carcinoma of the oral cavity rarely harbours oncogenic human papillomavirus. Oral Oncol 2011;47(8): 698–701.

149. Zhang ZY, Sdek P, Cao J, et al. Human papillomavirus type 16 and 18 DNA in oral squamous cell carcinoma and normal mucosa. Int J Oral Maxillofac Surg 2004;33(1):71–4.

150. Huang LW, Seow KM. Oral sex is a risk factor for human papillomavirus-associated nasopharyngeal carcinoma in husbands of women with cervical cancer. Gynecol Obstet Invest 2010;70(2):73–5.

151. Laantri N, Attaleb M, Kandil M, et al. Human papillomavirus detection in Moroccan patients with nasopharyngeal carcinoma. Infect Agent Cancer 2011;6(1):3.

152. Lo EJ, Bell D, Woo JS, et al. Human papillomavirus and WHO type I nasopharyngeal carcinoma. Laryngoscope 2010;120(10):1990–7.

153. Maxwell JH, Kumar B, Feng FY, et al. HPV-positive/p16-positive/EBV-negative nasopharyngeal carcinoma in white North Americans. Head Neck 2010;32(5): 562–7.

154. Mineta H, Ogino T, Amano HM, et al. Human papilloma virus (HPV) type 16 and 18 detected in head and neck squamous cell carcinoma. Anticancer Res 1998; 18(6B):4765–8.
155. Mirzamani N, Salehian P, Farhadi M, et al. Detection of EBV and HPV in nasopharyngeal carcinoma by in situ hybridization. Exp Mol Pathol 2006;81(3):231–4.
156. Singhi AD, Califano J, Westra WH. High-risk human papillomavirus in nasopharyngeal carcinoma. Head Neck 2012;34(2):213–8.
157. Bryan RL, Bevan IS, Crocker J, et al. Detection of HPV 6 and 11 in tumours of the upper respiratory tract using the polymerase chain reaction. Clin Otolaryngol Allied Sci 1990;15(2):177–80.
158. Kassim SK, Ibrahim SA, Eissa S, et al. Epstein-Barr virus, human papillomavirus, and flow cytometric cell cycle kinetics in nasopharyngeal carcinoma and inverted papilloma among Egyptian patients. Dis Markers 1998;14(2):113–20.
159. Krishna SM, James S, Kattoor J, et al. Human papilloma virus infection in Indian nasopharyngeal carcinomas in relation to the histology of tumour. Indian J Pathol Microbiol 2004;47(2):181–5.
160. Huang CC, Hsiao JR, Yang MW, et al. Human papilloma virus detection in neoplastic and non-neoplastic nasopharyngeal tissues in Taiwan. J Clin Pathol 2011;64(7):571–7.
161. Licitra L, Zigon G, Gatta G, et al. Human papillomavirus in HNSCC: a European epidemiologic perspective. Hematol Oncol Clin North Am 2008;22(6):1143, viii.
162. Hocking JS, Stein A, Conway EL, et al. Head and neck cancer in Australia between 1982 and 2005 show increasing incidence of potentially HPV-associated oropharyngeal cancers. Br J Cancer 2011;104(5):886–91.
163. Munoz N, Bosch FX, de Sanjose S, et al. Epidemiologic classification of human papillomavirus types associated with cervical cancer. N Engl J Med 2003; 348(6):518–27.
164. Schiffman M, Clifford G, Buonaguro FM. Classification of weakly carcinogenic human papillomavirus types: addressing the limits of epidemiology at the borderline. Infect Agent Cancer 2009;4:8.
165. Walboomers JM, Jacobs MV, Manos MM, et al. Human papillomavirus is a necessary cause of invasive cervical cancer worldwide. J Pathol 1999; 189(1):12–9.
166. Gillison ML, Lowy DR. A causal role for human papillomavirus in head and neck cancer. Lancet 2004;363(9420):1488–9.
167. Kreimer AR, Alberg AJ, Daniel R, et al. Oral human papillomavirus infection in adults is associated with sexual behavior and HIV serostatus. J Infect Dis 2004;189(4):686–98.
168. Kreimer AR, Villa A, Nyitray AG, et al. The epidemiology of oral HPV infection among a multinational sample of healthy men. Cancer Epidemiol Biomarkers Prev 2011;20(1):172–82.
169. Matsushita K, Sasagawa T, Miyashita M, et al. Oral and cervical human papillomavirus infection among female sex workers in Japan. Jpn J Infect Dis 2011; 64(1):34–9.
170. Parisi SG, Cruciani M, Scaggiante R, et al. Anal and oral human papillomavirus (HPV) infection in HIV infected subjects in Northern Italy: a longitudinal cohort study among men who have sex with men. BMC Infect Dis 2011;11(1):150.
171. Boonyanurak P, Panichakul S, Wilawan K. Prevalence of high-risk human papillomavirus infection (HPV) and correlation with postmenopausal hormonal therapy in Thai women aged more than 45 years old. J Med Assoc Thai 2010; 93(1):9–16.

172. Esquenazi D, Bussoloti Fl, Carvalho MG, et al. The frequency of human papillomavirus findings in normal oral mucosa of healthy people by PCR. Braz J Otorhinolaryngol 2010;76(1):78–84.
173. Termine N, Giovannelli L, Matranga D, et al. Low rate of oral human papillomavirus (HPV) infection in women screened for cervical HPV infection in Southern Italy: a cross-sectional study of 140 immunocompetent subjects. J Med Virol 2009;81(8):1438–43.
174. do Sacramento PR, Babeto E, Colombo J, et al. The prevalence of human papillomavirus in the oropharynx in healthy individuals in a Brazilian population. J Med Virol 2006;78(5):614–8.
175. D'Souza G, Agrawal Y, Halpern J, et al. Oral sexual behaviors associated with prevalent oral human papillomavirus infection. J Infect Dis 2009;199(9):1263–9.
176. Smith EM, Ritchie JM, Yankowitz J, et al. HPV prevalence and concordance in the cervix and oral cavity of pregnant women. Infect Dis Obstet Gynecol 2004;12(2):45–56.
177. Smith EM, Swarnavel S, Ritchie JM, et al. Prevalence of human papillomavirus in the oral cavity/oropharynx in a large population of children and adolescents. Pediatr Infect Dis J 2007;26(9):836–40.
178. Summersgill KF, Smith EM, Levy BT, et al. Human papillomavirus in the oral cavities of children and adolescents. Oral Surg Oral Med Oral Pathol Oral Radiol Endod 2001;91(1):62–9.
179. Kreimer AR, Bhatia RK, Messeguer AL, et al. Oral human papillomavirus in healthy individuals: a systematic review of the literature. Sex Transm Dis 2010;37(6):386–91.
180. D'Souza G, Fakhry C, Sugar EA, et al. Six-month natural history of oral versus cervical human papillomavirus infection. Int J Cancer 2007;121(1):143–50.
181. Huh WK. Human papillomavirus infection: a concise review of natural history. Obstet Gynecol 2009;114(1):139–43.
182. Insinga RP, Dasbach EJ, Elbasha EH. Epidemiologic natural history and clinical management of human papillomavirus (HPV) disease: a critical and systematic review of the literature in the development of an HPV dynamic transmission model. BMC Infect Dis 2009;9:119.
183. Kurose K, Terai M, Soedarsono N, et al. Low prevalence of HPV infection and its natural history in normal oral mucosa among volunteers on Miyako Island, Japan. Oral Surg Oral Med Oral Pathol Oral Radiol Endod 2004;98(1):91–6.
184. Rintala M, Grenman S, Puranen M, et al. Natural history of oral papillomavirus infections in spouses: a prospective Finnish HPV Family Study. J Clin Virol 2006;35(1):89–94.
185. Rintala MA, Grenman SE, Jarvenkyla ME, et al. High-risk types of human papillomavirus (HPV) DNA in oral and genital mucosa of infants during their first 3 years of life: experience from the Finnish HPV Family Study. Clin Infect Dis 2005;41(12):1728–33.
186. D'Souza G, Kluz N, Stammer E, et al. Oral HPV prevalence and persistence among high risk young adults. 27th International Papillomavirus Conference and Clinical Workshop. Berlin, September 17–22, 2011. Poster P-16.36.
187. Benard VB, Johnson CJ, Thompson TD, et al. Examining the association between socioeconomic status and potential human papillomavirus-associated cancers. Cancer 2008;113(Suppl 10):2910–8.
188. Ang KK, Harris J, Wheeler R, et al. Human papillomavirus and survival of patients with oropharyngeal cancer. N Engl J Med 2010;363(1):24–35.

189. Beachler DC, D'Souza G. Nuances in the changing epidemiology of head and neck cancer. Oncology 2010;24(10):924–6.
190. Ryerson AB, Peters ES, Coughlin SS, et al. Burden of potentially human papillomavirus-associated cancers of the oropharynx and oral cavity in the US, 1998-2003. Cancer 2008;113(Suppl 10):2901–9.
191. Rajkumar T, Sridhar H, Balaram P, et al. Oral cancer in Southern India: the influence of body size, diet, infections and sexual practices. Eur J Cancer Prev 2003;12(2):135–43.
192. Rosenquist K, Wennerberg J, Schildt EB, et al. Oral status, oral infections and some lifestyle factors as risk factors for oral and oropharyngeal squamous cell carcinoma. A population-based case-control study in southern Sweden. Acta Otolaryngol 2005;125(12):1327–36.
193. Heck JE, Berthiller J, Vaccarella S, et al. Sexual behaviours and the risk of head and neck cancers: a pooled analysis in the International Head and Neck Cancer Epidemiology (INHANCE) consortium. Int J Epidemiol 2010;39(1):166–81.
194. D'Souza G, Zhang HH, D'Souza WD, et al. Moderate predictive value of demographic and behavioral characteristics for a diagnosis of HPV16-positive and HPV16-negative head and neck cancer. Oral Oncol 2010;46(2):100–4.
195. Maxwell JH, Kumar B, Feng FY, et al. Tobacco use in human papillomavirus-positive advanced oropharynx cancer patients related to increased risk of distant metastases and tumor recurrence. Clin Cancer Res 2010;16(4):1226–35.
196. Schrank TP, Han Y, Weiss H, et al. Case-matching analysis of head and neck squamous cell carcinoma in racial and ethnic minorities in the United States–possible role for human papillomavirus in survival disparities. Head Neck 2011;33(1):45–53.
197. Ringstrom E, Peters E, Hasegawa M, et al. Human papillomavirus type 16 and squamous cell carcinoma of the head and neck. Clin Cancer Res 2002;8(10): 3187–92.
198. Fukushima K, Ogura H, Watanabe S, et al. Human papillomavirus type 16 DNA detected by the polymerase chain reaction in non-cancer tissues of the head and neck. Eur Arch Otorhinolaryngol 1994;251(2):109–12.
199. Anaya-Saavedra G, Ramirez-Amador V, Irigoyen-Camacho ME, et al. High association of human papillomavirus infection with oral cancer: a case-control study. Arch Med Res 2008;39(2):189–97.
200. Balaram P, Nalinakumari KR, Abraham E, et al. Human papillomaviruses in 91 oral cancers from Indian betel quid chewers–high prevalence and multiplicity of infections. Int J Cancer 1995;61(4):450–4.
201. Campisi G, Giovannelli L, Calvino F, et al. HPV infection in relation to OSCC histological grading and TNM stage. Evaluation by traditional statistics and fuzzy logic model. Oral Oncol 2006;42(6):638–45.
202. Cunningham LL Jr, Pagano GM, Li M, et al. Overexpression of p16INK4 is a reliable marker of human papillomavirus-induced oral high-grade squamous dysplasia. Oral Surg Oral Med Oral Pathol Oral Radiol Endod 2006;102(1):77–81.
203. da Silva CE, da Silva ID, Cerri A, et al. Prevalence of human papillomavirus in squamous cell carcinoma of the tongue. Oral Surg Oral Med Oral Pathol Oral Radiol Endod 2007;104(4):497–500.
204. D'Costa J, Saranath D, Dedhia P, et al. Detection of HPV-16 genome in human oral cancers and potentially malignant lesions from India. Oral Oncol 1998; 34(5):413–20.
205. Hafkamp HC, Speel EJ, Haesevoets A, et al. A subset of head and neck squamous cell carcinomas exhibits integration of HPV 16/18 DNA and overexpression of

p16INK4A and p53 in the absence of mutations in p53 exons 5-8. Int J Cancer 2003;107(3):394–400.

206. Ibieta BR, Lizano M, Fras-Mendivil M, et al. Human papilloma virus in oral squamous cell carcinoma in a Mexican population. Oral Surg Oral Med Oral Pathol Oral Radiol Endod 2005;99(3):311–5.

207. Ishibashi M, Kishino M, Sato S, et al. The prevalence of human papillomavirus in oral premalignant lesions and squamous cell carcinoma in comparison to cervical lesions used as a positive control. Int J Clin Oncol 2011;16(6):646–53.

208. Jalouli J, Ibrahim SO, Sapkota D, et al. Presence of human papilloma virus, herpes simplex virus and Epstein-Barr virus DNA in oral biopsies from Sudanese patients with regard to toombak use. J Oral Pathol Med 2010;39(8):599–604.

209. Joo YH, Jung CK, Sun DI, et al. High-risk human papillomavirus and cervical lymph node metastasis in patients with oropharyngeal cancer. Head Neck 2012;34(1):10–4.

210. Koppikar P, deVilliers EM, Mulherkar R. Identification of human papillomaviruses in tumors of the oral cavity in an Indian community. Int J Cancer 2005;113(6): 946–50.

211. Kozomara R, Jovic N, Magic Z, et al. p53 mutations and human papillomavirus infection in oral squamous cell carcinomas: correlation with overall survival. J Craniomaxillofac Surg 2005;33(5):342–8.

212. Lee SY, Cho NH, Choi EC, et al. Relevance of human papilloma virus (HPV) infection to carcinogenesis of oral tongue cancer. Int J Oral Maxillofac Surg 2010;39(7):678–83.

213. Liang XH, Lewis J, Foote R, et al. Prevalence and significance of human papillomavirus in oral tongue cancer: the Mayo Clinic experience. J Oral Maxillofac Surg 2008;66(9):1875–80.

214. Lohavanichbutr P, Houck J, Fan W, et al. Genomewide gene expression profiles of HPV-positive and HPV-negative oropharyngeal cancer: potential implications for treatment choices. Arch Otolaryngol Head Neck Surg 2009; 135(2):180–8.

215. Machado J, Reis PP, Zhang T, et al. Low prevalence of human papillomavirus in oral cavity carcinomas. Head Neck Oncol 2010;2:6.

216. Mao EJ, Schwartz SM, Daling JR, et al. Human papilloma viruses and p53 mutations in normal pre-malignant and malignant oral epithelia. Int J Cancer 1996; 69(2):152–8.

217. Mendelsohn AH, Lai CK, Shintaku IP, et al. Histopathologic findings of HPV and p16 positive HNSCC. Laryngoscope 2010;120(9):1788–94.

218. Nagpal JK, Patnaik S, Das BR. Prevalence of high-risk human papilloma virus types and its association with P53 codon 72 polymorphism in tobacco addicted oral squamous cell carcinoma (OSCC) patients of Eastern India. Int J Cancer 2002;97(5):649–53.

219. Nemes JA, Deli L, Nemes Z, et al. Expression of p16(INK4A), p53, and Rb proteins are independent from the presence of human papillomavirus genes in oral squamous cell carcinoma. Oral Surg Oral Med Oral Pathol Oral Radiol Endod 2006;102(3):344–52.

220. Oliveira LR, Ribeiro-Silva A, Ramalho LN, et al. HPV infection in Brazilian oral squamous cell carcinoma patients and its correlation with clinicopathological outcomes. Mol Med Report 2008;1(1):123–9.

221. Oliveira MC, Soares RC, Pinto LP, et al. High-risk human papillomavirus (HPV) is not associated with p53 and bcl-2 expression in oral squamous cell carcinomas. Auris Nasus Larynx 2009;36(4):450–6.

222. Premoli-De-Percoco G, Ramirez JL. High risk human papillomavirus in oral squamous carcinoma: evidence of risk factors in a Venezuelan rural population. Preliminary report. J Oral Pathol Med 2001;30(6):355–61.

223. Ragin CC, Taioli E, Weissfeld JL, et al. 11q13 amplification status and human papillomavirus in relation to p16 expression defines two distinct etiologies of head and neck tumours. Br J Cancer 2006;95(10):1432–8.

224. Ribeiro KB, Levi JE, Pawlita M, et al. Low human papillomavirus prevalence in head and neck cancer: results from two large case-control studies in high-incidence regions. Int J Epidemiol 2011;40(2):489–502.

225. Riethdorf S, Friedrich RE, Ostwald C, et al. p53 gene mutations and HPV infection in primary head and neck squamous cell carcinomas do not correlate with overall survival: a long-term follow-up study. J Oral Pathol Med 1997;26(7): 315–21.

226. Rivero ER, Nunes FD. HPV in oral squamous cell carcinomas of a Brazilian population: amplification by PCR. Braz Oral Res 2006;20(1):21–4.

227. Saini R, Tang TH, Zain RB, et al. Significant association of high-risk human papillomavirus (HPV) but not of p53 polymorphisms with oral squamous cell carcinomas in Malaysia. J Cancer Res Clin Oncol 2011;137(2):311–20.

228. Scapoli L, Palmieri A, Rubini C, et al. Low prevalence of human papillomavirus in squamous-cell carcinoma limited to oral cavity proper. Mod Pathol 2009;22(3): 366–72.

229. Simonato LE, Garcia JF, Sundefeld ML, et al. Detection of HPV in mouth floor squamous cell carcinoma and its correlation with clinicopathologic variables, risk factors and survival. J Oral Pathol Med 2008;37(10):593–8.

230. Smith EM, Rubenstein LM, Hoffman H, et al. Human papillomavirus, p16 and p53 expression associated with survival of head and neck cancer. Infect Agent Cancer 2010;5:4.

231. Soares RC, Oliveira MC, Souza LB, et al. Human papillomavirus in oral squamous cells carcinoma in a population of 75 Brazilian patients. Am J Otolaryngol 2007;28(6):397–400.

232. St Guily JL, Jacquard AC, Pretet JL, et al. Human papillomavirus genotype distribution in oropharynx and oral cavity cancer in France–the EDiTH VI study. J Clin Virol 2011;51(2):100–4.

233. Sugiyama M, Bhawal UK, Dohmen T, et al. Detection of human papillomavirus-16 and HPV-18 DNA in normal, dysplastic, and malignant oral epithelium. Oral Surg Oral Med Oral Pathol Oral Radiol Endod 2003; 95(5):594–600.

234. Tang X, Jia L, Ouyang J, et al. Comparative study of HPV prevalence in Japanese and North-east Chinese oral carcinoma. J Oral Pathol Med 2003;32(7): 393–8.

235. Tsuhako K, Nakazato I, Miyagi J, et al. Comparative study of oral squamous cell carcinoma in Okinawa, Southern Japan and Sapporo in Hokkaido, Northern Japan; with special reference to human papillomavirus and Epstein-Barr virus infection. J Oral Pathol Med 2000;29(2):70–9.

236. Weiss D, Koopmann M, Rudack C. Prevalence and impact on clinicopathological characteristics of human papillomavirus-16 DNA in cervical lymph node metastases of head and neck squamous cell carcinoma. Head Neck 2011; 33(6):856–62.

237. Yamakawa-Kakuta Y, Kawamata H, Doi Y, et al. Does the expression of HPV 16/18 E6/E7 in head and neck squamous cell carcinomas relate to their clinicopathological characteristics? Int J Oncol 2009;35(5):983–8.

238. Gungor A, Cincik H, Baloglu H, et al. Human papilloma virus prevalence in laryngeal squamous cell carcinoma. J Laryngol Otol 2007;121(8):772–4.
239. Rodrigo JP, Gonzalez MV, Lazo PS, et al. Genetic alterations in squamous cell carcinomas of the hypopharynx with correlations to clinicopathological features. Oral Oncol 2002;38(4):357–63.

Detection of Human Papillomavirus in Clinical Samples

William H. Westra, MD[a,b,c,*]

KEYWORDS

- Oropharyngeal carcinoma • Squamous cell carcinoma of the head and neck
- In situ hybridization • Hybrid capture 2 • p16 immunohistochemistry

KEY POINTS

- Identification of human papillomavirus (HPV) in squamous cell carcinomas of the head and neck is rapidly becoming a means of tracking the presence and progress of disease relating to all aspects of patient care, including prognosis, tumor staging (ie, identifying site of tumor origin), and selection of patients who are most likely to benefit from tailored therapeutic options.
- At present, there is no standard approach for HPV testing of clinical samples. The challenge for the oncologic community is to implement standardized HPV testing using a method that is highly accurate, technically feasible, and cost effective.
- The use of p16 immunohistochemical staining is acceptable as a method of HPV detection, provided it is used and interpreted in a defined context that takes into account certain anatomic factors, histologic findings, and staining characteristics.
- The development of detection assays that are optimized for cytologic samples will lead to more widespread implementation of HPV testing and may obviate tissue acquisition and processing.

INTRODUCTION

Squamous cell carcinoma of the head and neck (HNSCC) has long been regarded as a monotonous disease entity. Important distinctions between anatomic subsites and natural histories have largely been ignored, given the histopathologic uniformity and response to treatment. Recent studies suggest considerable differences between some HNSCCs that go beyond variations related to tumor subsite and stage. In

The author has no relevant financial or commercial relationships to disclose.
[a] Department of Pathology, The Johns Hopkins Medical Institutions, Baltimore, MD, USA;
[b] Department of Oncology, The Johns Hopkins Medical Institutions, Baltimore, MD, USA;
[c] Department of Otolaryngology–Head and Neck Surgery, The Johns Hopkins Medical Institutions, Baltimore, MD, USA
* Corresponding author. The Johns Hopkins Hospital, 401 North Broadway, Weinberg 2242, Baltimore, MD 21231-2410.
E-mail address: wwestra@jhmi.edu

Otolaryngol Clin N Am 45 (2012) 765–777
doi:10.1016/j.otc.2012.04.001
0030-6665/12/$ – see front matter © 2012 Elsevier Inc. All rights reserved.

particular, a subset of HNSCCs, which is associated with the human papillomavirus (HPV), has emerged as a form of HNSCC with an epidemiologic, demographic, histopathologic, and clinical profile that deviates from the profile of conventional non-HPV–related HNSCC.[1,2] HPV-associated cancers tend to occur more frequently in younger men, and tobacco smoking does not seem to be a strong cofactor in the development of these tumors.[3,4] These cancers most frequently occur in the oropharynx,[2,5] tend to exhibit a nonkeratinizing basaloid morphology,[6,7] and are associated with improved clinical outcomes.[2,8–10] In effect, recognition of this association with HPV amounts to the identification of a new and distinct disease entity.

WHY IS HPV TESTING IMPORTANT?

Until recently, clinicians have not been able to rely on prognostic markers other than tumor staging in their care of patients with HNSCC. Although numerous studies have addressed the prognostic relevance of cell proliferation (eg, Ki67, proliferating cell nuclear antigen), p53 immunohistochemical staining, apoptosis, aneuploidy, epidermal growth factor receptor overexpression, and various other markers of biological activity, none of these markers have proved consistently reliable across multiple studies. None of these markers are currently used as a routine part of pathologic evaluation for patient care. The absence of reliable prognostic markers has been offset to some degree by HPV testing. The detection of HPV in HNSCCs has recently emerged as a powerful biomarker, indicating a more favorable clinical outcome. Patients with HPV-positive tumors have a lower risk of tumor progression and death than patients with HPV-negative tumors.[2,8–10] Accordingly, inclusion of HPV status as a parameter for emerging molecular staging systems is compelling, and routine HPV assessment will soon become part of the standard pathologic evaluation of all oropharyngeal carcinomas. Both the College of American Pathologists and the American Joint Committee on Cancer have recently recommended routine HPV testing as part of the standard pathologic evaluation of resected oropharyngeal squamous cell carcinomas for the purpose of molecular tumor staging.[11,12]

The value of HPV testing is by no means confined to mere prognostication in patients with HNSCC. A study that analyzed the motivations for HPV testing in the clinical arena found that HPV testing was often initiated by the pathologist to help resolve difficult diagnostic dilemmas.[13] For example, HPV testing of cervical lymph node metastases is a highly effective strategy for localizing the site of origin in those patients who present with neck metastases in the absence of an obvious primary tumor. In these patients, the detection of HPV in a lymph node metastasis is a reliable predictor of oropharyngeal origin (**Fig. 1**).[14,15] Similarly, HPV status can be used to clarify second primary or metastatic disease in those patients with HNSCC who subsequently develop squamous cell carcinoma in their lungs.[16] In some instances, HPV status can inform the differential diagnosis, such as squamous-lined cysts of the lateral neck, where an HPV-positive cystic metastasis can easily be confused with an inflamed branchial cleft cyst.[17]

As more is understood of the unique natural history of HPV-positive HNSCC, from viral infection to viral persistence to viral-induced malignant transformation, applications for HPV testing will undoubtedly continue to increase. The detection of HPV is emerging as a valid biomarker for discerning the presence and progress of disease, encompassing all aspects of patient care:

- Early cancer detection.[18]
- More accurate tumor staging.[14,15]

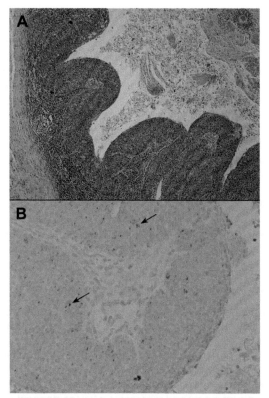

Fig. 1. (*A*) Metastatic cystic squamous cell carcinoma involving a level II cervical lymph node in a patient without a known primary tumor (hematoxylin-eosin, original magnification ×10). (*B*) Although the primary tumor is clinically occult, the detection of HPV in the metastatic carcinoma strongly suggests that the tumor originated from the oropharynx (HPV-16 DNA in situ hybridization, *arrows* point to the hybridization signals within the tumor cell nuclei) (HPV-16 in situ hybridization, original magnification ×40).

- Selection of patients most likely to benefit from specific treatments.[19]
- Posttreatment tumor surveillance.[20,21]

As for clinical research, study design and data analysis must incorporate HPV status into the next generation of clinical trials. Knowledge of HPV status is compulsory for meaningful comparison of treatment responses in patients enrolled in these trials. The direction of current clinical trials in which patient selection for specific therapies is predicated based on HPV tumor status dramatically heightens the stakes for accurate HPV detection.

WHEN IS HPV TESTING APPROPRIATE?
Site-Directed HPV Testing

HPV is not evenly distributed across all anatomic subsites in HNSCC. Instead, HPV infection is strongly correlated with oropharyngeal location, particularly the palatine and lingual tonsils.[2,5,22] This correlation is so strong that the detection of HPV in an adjacent oropharyngeal site raises consideration of direct local extension from an oropharyngeal primary carcinoma.[23] This preferential targeting likely reflects complex biological interactions between HPV and the highly specialized lymphoepithelial lining of the tonsillar crypts.[24] Based on the localization of HPV-related HNSCC to the oropharynx, directives for routine HPV testing are generally restricted to those carcinomas arising from this specific anatomic subsite.[11,12] Although HPV positivity is sometimes reported in HNSCCs arising outside the oropharynx, such as the sinonasal tract,[25] expanding the scope of routine HPV testing is not warranted until well-designed studies establish a clear relationship between HPV infection at these nonoropharyngeal sites and a distinct natural history, including treatment responses.

HPV Testing of Lymph Node Metastases

In malignant transformation of the tonsillar epithelium, HPV does not act through a "hit-and-run" mechanism whereby its role is transient and limited to the initiation of tumorigenesis. Instead, the presence of HPV persists, and it is just as readily detected in metastatic implants as in the corresponding primary cancers.[5] Consequently, a lymph node metastasis is quite suitable as a substrate for HPV testing, obviating additional tissue acquisition in those patients with small or even occult primary cancers.

HOW IS HPV DETECTED IN CLINICAL SAMPLES?
A Summary of the Biology of HPV as an Oncologic Agent

Various strategies are currently available for HPV analysis. An objective evaluation of these assays, including a comparison of their strengths and weaknesses, requires a fundamental understanding of the way HPV induces malignant transformation of the tonsillar epithelium, particularly its interaction with key components of the retinoblastoma (Rb) tumor suppressor gene pathway.

The p16 tumor suppressor gene, located on chromosome 9p21, is a member of the INK4 class of cell cycle inhibitors and represents a key component of the Rb pathway. Binding of the p16 tumor suppressor gene product with cyclin-dependent kinases 4 and 6 blocks its interaction with D-type cyclins, maintains the Rb gene in a hypophosphorylated state that binds the E2F transcription factor, and, in turn, prevents cell-cycle progression.[26] In conventional (ie, non-HPV related) HNSCC, the p16 tumor suppressor gene is inactivated by various genetic and nongenetic (eg, promoter hypermethylation) modifications, such that the expression of its protein product is lost or dramatically diminished.[27] By contrast, integration of high-risk HPV into the host genome is associated with upregulation of the p16 tumor suppressor gene product. Integration of HPV results in the deletion of the viral E2 gene promoter, causing transcription of E6 and E7.[28] Binding of the E7 oncoprotein to the Rb protein leads to Rb protein degradation and, presumably, the compensatory overexpression of both cytoplasmic and nuclear p16 proteins in HPV-infected tumor cells.

Given the capacity to target and disrupt the Rb tumor suppressor gene pathway, HPV detection strategies focus on the detection of:

1. The actual presence of HPV DNA
2. Postintegration transcription of viral E6 and/or E7 messenger RNA (mRNA)
3. The viral oncoproteins E6 and E7
4. Altered expression of cellular proteins, such as overexpression of the p16 protein.

The Morphology of HPV-Related HNSCC

HPV-related HNSCC has a consistent microscopic appearance that diverges from the typical morphology of non-HPV–related HNSCC (**Table 1**).[7] Although the documentation of HPV status requires HPV testing, microscopic findings can successfully guide

Table 1
Contrasting histologic features of conventional HNSCC and HPV-related oropharyngeal carcinoma

Histologic Features	Conventional Squamous Cell Carcinoma	HPV-Related Oropharyngeal Squamous Cell Carcinoma
Origin	Surface epithelium	Reticulated epithelium of tonsillar crypts
Surface dysplasia	Present	Absent
Growth pattern	Irregular cords and nests	Sheets and rounded lobules
Desmoplasia	Prominent	Often absent
Keratinization	Prominent	Minimal or absent
Differentiation	Moderately differentiated	Immature and basaloid (often interpreted as poorly differentiated)
Tumor-infiltrating lymphocytes	Usually absent	Often present

the implementation and interpretation of HPV analysis. Unlike most conventional HNSCCs, HPV-related HNSCCs do not typically arise from the surface epithelium showing a background of dysplastic changes, do not infiltrate as irregular cords and nests of cells that elicit a prominent desmoplastic stromal reaction, and do not show prominent cytoplasmic keratinization. Instead, HPV-related HNSCCs characteristically arise from the specialized reticulated epithelium of tonsillar crypts in the absence of dysplastic (ie, premalignant) changes in the surface squamous epithelium, often grow as rounded nests and lobules, are often permeated by infiltrating lymphocytes, and have tumor cells that display a high nuclear to cytoplasmic ratio, minimal keratinization, and a highly immature or basaloid appearance (**Fig. 2**). The likelihood that the tumor is HPV related is very high when these features are present and well developed in oropharyngeal carcinoma.

Gold Standard HPV Testing

The ultimate value of any HPV detection strategy lies in its ability to both recognize the presence of HPV and discern its potential as a driving force of tumorigenesis. For example, a given assay may be highly sensitive in its ability to detect trace amounts of HPV but may have no clinical value if it cannot differentiate an incidental virus (eg, passenger virus or viral contaminant) from an active oncologic agent. Evidence for transcriptional activation of the viral oncoproteins E6 and E7 is generally regarded as the gold standard for clinically relevant HPV. In the absence of reliable immunohistochemical probes for E6 and E7 proteins, detection of E6/E7 mRNA is the current standard by which the sensitivities and specificities of all other detection assays are measured. Until recently, detection of E6/E7 mRNA expression has required the extraction of RNA from fresh or frozen tissues followed by polymerase chain reaction (PCR) amplification of viral RNA. Although the transfer of this technique to formalin-fixed and paraffin-embedded (FFPE) tissues has greatly expanded its application to clinical samples, the technique remains technically challenging and its use is mainly restricted to the research laboratory.

The ongoing challenge in detecting HPV has been to reproduce the accuracy and reliability of the PCR E6/E7 mRNA assay using techniques that are easier and commonplace to the diagnostic pathologic laboratory. In studies that have used this gold standard to evaluate the effectiveness of other detection strategies, p16 immunohistochemical staining (described later) has been found to be highly sensitive but

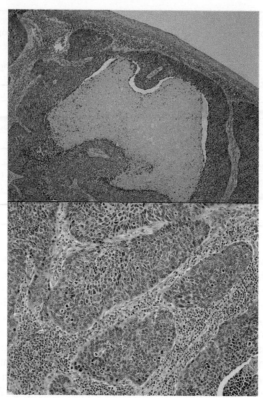

Fig. 2. HPV-related squamous cell carcinoma of the tonsil. These tumors tend to fill and expand the tonsillar crypts, often forming large lobules with central cystic necrosis. The overlying surface epithelium is intact and without dysplastic changes (*upper panel*) (hematoxylin-eosin, original magnification ×4). At higher power, the tumor infiltrates as rounded basaloid nests that lack significant keratinization and are surrounded by a lymphoid stroma (*lower panel*) (hematoxylin-eosin, original magnification ×20).

not entirely specific, whereas HPV DNA in situ hybridization (ISH) has been found to be highly specific but not entirely sensitive in the detection of HPV.[29]

Methods of HPV Detection

At present, there is no standard approach for HPV testing of clinical samples. Methods of HPV testing vary considerably across laboratories, reflecting the biases and tendencies of individual investigators and the cost-to-benefit ratio of each technique (**Table 2**).[30] Detection strategies vary not just in design but also in their detection targets. These targets have included HPV DNA, HPV RNA, viral oncoproteins, cellular proteins, and HPV-specific serum antibodies. Detection methods must be accurate, technically feasible, and cost effective for widespread implementation in the clinical arena. For example, detection of mRNA E6/E7 transcripts may be the gold standard for HPV detection, but the increased demand for expertise and processing of complex tissue (eg, microdissection of fresh frozen tissue) limits its application as a routine diagnostic tool. At the other extreme, immunohistochemical staining for viral proteins is relatively simple and inexpensive, but the performance of this approach has been too inconsistent to be used as a reliable detection method.

Table 2
Comparison of HPV detection methods

Method	Advantages	Disadvantages
HPV DNA		
Consensus and type-specific PCR	High sensitivity	Inability to discern clinically relevant infections from irrelevant infections
Real-time PCR	High sensitivity and specificity, estimation of viral load	Requires complex tissue processing (eg, microdissection, DNA extraction)
ISH	Optimized for fixed tissues, visualization of viral distribution, highly specific	Reduced specificity at low viral load
Hybrid capture 2	Can be applied to cytologic samples, no need for specimen processing	Further studies are needed to determine overall sensitivity and specificity
HPV RNA		
Reverse transcriptase PCR	Highly sensitive, highly specific	Limited to fresh frozen tissue
HPV proteins		
E6/E7 immunohistochemistry	Visualization of oncoprotein expression	Poor performance
Cellular proteins		
p16 immunohistochemical staining	Optimized for fixed tissues, highly sensitive, strong correlation with HPV integration	Low specificity
Serum antibodies		
Anti-HPV protein antibodies	Minimally invasive, no tissue requirement	Marker of lifetime cumulative exposure to HPV, low sensitivity and specificity as cancer marker

Data from Robinson M, Sloan P, Shaw R. Refining the diagnosis of oropharyngeal squamous cell carcinoma using human papillomavirus testing. Oral Oncol 2010;46:492–6.

At present, most diagnostic laboratories that perform routine testing of clinical samples use 1 of the 2 methods for HPV detection:

1. PCR-based amplification
2. DNA ISH.

PCR-Based Amplification

PCR-based amplification of HPV DNA is a target amplification technique that is capable of amplifying trace DNA sequences in a biological sample that contains heterogeneous cell types. The primers used can be specific for individual HPV types or a target consensus sequence shared by multiple HPV types. When used as a nonquantitative technique, it provides no information regarding the abundance of a particular DNA species.

DNA ISH

DNA ISH is a signal amplification technique that uses labeled DNA probes complementary to targeted viral DNA sequences. The DNA probes may hybridize to HPV type–specific DNA sequences or a consensus sequence shared by multiple HPV types or may be mixed in a single reaction to cover an extended range of HPV types (ie, probe cocktail). The performance of these 2 techniques is comparable, although a direct comparison suggests that DNA ISH may be a more practical tool for diagnostic purposes:

1. The development of nonfluorescent chromogens now allows visualization of DNA hybridization using conventional light microscopy.
2. The introduction of various signal amplification steps has significantly improved the sensitivity of ISH, even to the level of detecting one viral copy per cell.
3. The adaptation of ISH to FFPE tissues has made this technique compatible with standard tissue processing procedures and, consequently, readily transferable to most surgical pathology laboratories.
4. Direct visualization of viral distribution in the nuclei of tumor cells more reliably differentiates biologically relevant HPV infection from passenger virus or even a viral contaminant.

Immunostaining for p16

Immunostaining for the p16 protein has been regarded as a practical alternative or complimentary procedure for HPV testing of oropharyngeal cancers based on the high correlation between HPV detection and p16 overexpression in recent studies (**Fig. 3**).[5,31,32] The simplicity, low cost, and high sensitivity of p16 immunohistochemical staining have prompted the consideration of replacing more intensive HPV DNA ISH

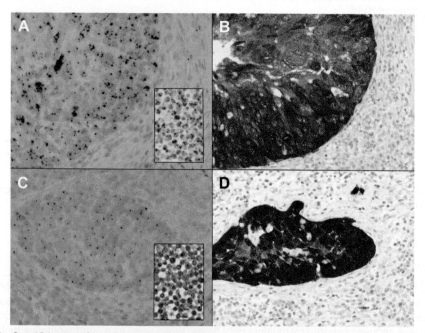

Fig. 3. p16 immunohistochemical staining is a reliable surrogate marker for the presence of HPV and reflects viral tissue distribution as determined by HPV-16 DNA ISH. p16 staining is strong and diffuse (*B* and *D*, original magnification ×40) even when the number of hybridization signals within the tumor nuclei vary (*A* and *C*, original magnification ×40). The insets show the positive cell line controls, CaSki (containing approximately 500 integrated copies of HPV-16) (*inset, A*) and SiHa (containing 1–2 integrated copies of HPV-16) (*inset, C*).

and PCR-based methods with this straightforward diagnostic approach. However, the mechanistic link between HPV DNA integration and p16 expression is neither direct nor exclusive. The Rb gene may be inactivated by mechanisms other than E7 oncoprotein expression, yet resulting in high levels of p16 expression.[33] Consequently, high levels of p16 proteins levels may be encountered in some carcinomas that are unrelated to high-risk HPV. To be truly useful as a surrogate marker of HPV infection, the interpretation of p16 immunohistochemical staining must be informed by various histologic, anatomic, and clinical considerations, as indicated in **Box 1**.

FUTURE DIRECTIONS IN HPV TESTING
Emerging Novel Techniques

The ultimate goal of any developing technology for HPV detection in clinical samples is to approach the gold standard for sensitivity and specificity while maximizing

---

Box 1
Guidelines for the interpretation of p16 immunohistochemical staining as a surrogate marker of HPV infection in HNSCC

Pattern and Intensity of p16 Immunohistochemical Staining

- p16 immunohistochemical staining may substitute for HPV testing when strong staining is present in the nucleus and cytoplasm of the tumor cells throughout all or most of the tumor. Focal or weak staining should be supported by HPV testing (either by in situ or PCR-based methods).

Anatomic Site of Tumor Origin

- Although the sensitivity and specificity of p16 staining as a marker of HPV infection is sufficiently high to serve as a reliable test for squamous cell carcinomas of oropharyngeal origin, these values are either unknown or unacceptably low for HNSCCs arising in nonoropharyngeal sites.
  - o p16 immunochemical staining may substitute for HPV testing in patients with carcinomas of known oropharyngeal origin.
  - o For lymph node metastases, p16 immunohistochemical staining may substitute for HPV testing in patients with a known oropharyngeal primary carcinoma or an oropharyngeal mass.
  - o For lymph node metastases in patients with an occult primary carcinoma, p16 immunohistochemical staining may substitute for HPV detection when the lymph node metastasis (1) involves a cervical lymph node in levels II to IV, (2) exhibits cystic degeneration, and (3) demonstrates characteristic HPV-associated histomorphology.

Tumor Histomorphology

- HPV-related oropharyngeal carcinomas demonstrate a consistent histomorphology (see **Table 1**). p16 immunohistochemical staining may substitute for HPV detection in oropharyngeal carcinomas that conform to this histology.
  - o Further HPV testing should be performed in patients with p16-negative oropharyngeal carcinomas that exhibit classic HPV-related histomorphology.
  - o Further HPV testing should be performed in patients with p16-positive oropharyngeal carcinomas that do not exhibit classic HPV morphology.

Clinical Indications

- At present, p16 immunohistochemical staining is used primarily as a prognostic indicator for patients with oropharyngeal carcinoma. Any expanded clinical role for HPV detection, such as selection criterion for HPV-specific therapies (eg, therapeutic vaccines, de-escalation protocols), may necessitate more stringent detection methods.

efficiency, simplicity, reproducibility, and transferability to the routine diagnostic laboratory. Although the documentation of transcriptionally active HPV in tumor cells is the most direct and compelling evidence of HPV-related tumorigenesis, the detection of E6/E7 transcripts has technical challenges, requiring RNA extraction from fresh frozen tissue as a substrate for PCR-based techniques. Furthermore, PCR-based techniques do not allow for direct visualization of the tissue distribution in transcriptionally active virus. The recent development of RNA ISH probes complementary to E6/E7 mRNA now permits direct visualization of viral transcripts in routinely processed tissues.[34] It is ideal to test for HPV E6/E7 transcripts using RNA ISH because it confirms the presence of integrated and transcriptionally active virus, permits the direct visualization of viral transcripts in tumor cells of tissue sections, is technically feasible, and has been strongly correlated with improved patient outcomes.[34]

HPV Testing of Cytologic Specimens

In all probability, the widespread implementation of HPV testing in the clinical arena will not move forward with much momentum until methods are developed for the testing of cytologic specimens, including fine-needle aspirations of neck metastases and brushings of primary tumors. The use of aspirated cells as a substrate for HPV assessment could facilitate the diagnosis of an HNSCC, direct the search for its site of origin, predict clinical outcome, and select patients who are most likely to benefit from immunology-based therapy; all while abrogating the need for tissue acquisition via a more aggressive surgical procedure. The few studies that have addressed HPV testing of cytologic samples have primarily tried to adapt tissue-targeted approaches (eg, p16 immunohistochemical staining and HPV ISH) to archived cytologic specimens.[15,35–37] In most instances, HPV testing of cytologic specimens is restricted to a small subset of cases in which ample cellular material is available for the construction of cell blocks. More broad-based applications await the development of novel strategies that can be applied to aspirated cells without the need for high cellularity and complex specimen processing.

In a recent feasibility study, the hybrid capture 2 assay, a commercially available microplate analysis, approved by the US Food and Drug Administration for the detection of HPV DNA as part of cervical cancer screening,[38,39] was found to reliably determine the HPV status of HNSCCs based on evaluation of cytologic specimens.[40] The hybrid capture 2 assay has several advantages over other methods of HPV detection:

1. Specimens can be easily collected without the need for tumor microdissection, formalin fixation, or specimen processing of any kind.
2. The liquid-phase medium serves not only as a transport medium but also as a storage medium, such that there is no need for rapid specimen transport to minimize specimen degradation.
3. Automation ensures reproducibility and provides the capacity for handling increasing volumes of clinical samples.
4. Results that are obtained on the same day permit timely treatment decisions including study enrollment by eliminating HPV determination as a rate-limiting factor.
5. It is cost effective.
6. It can be applied to cytologic samples.

Confirmation of the hybrid capture 2 assay as a reliable and feasible means of HPV evaluation of cytologic samples awaits the findings of the assay's use in several prospectively evaluated patients with HNSCC.

SUMMARY

1. HNSCCs have long been regarded as a uniform disease entity. The oncogenic HPV, particularly type HPV-16, has now been established as a causative agent in up to 80% of oropharyngeal cancers. These HPV-positive HNSCCs differ from HPV-negative HNSCCs in important aspects, rendering the HNSCCs as a group that is much more heterogeneous than predicted, with a major subdivision occurring along the HPV status.
2. Determination of HPV status is important. The identification of HPV in HNSCC is rapidly becoming a means of tracking the presence and progress of disease relating to all aspects of patient care, including prognosis, tumor staging (ie, identifying site of tumor origin), and selection of patients who are most likely to benefit from tailored therapeutic options.
3. At present, there is no standard approach for the testing of HPV in clinical samples. The challenge for the oncologic community is to implement standardized HPV testing using a method that is highly accurate, technically feasible, and cost effective. This has been difficult, as each test is associated with its own unique strengths and weaknesses (see **Table 2**).
4. One detection method that is soaring in popularity is the immunohistochemical detection of the cellular protein p16. The use of p16 immunohistochemical staining is acceptable as a method of HPV detection, provided it is used and interpreted in a defined context that takes into account certain anatomic factors, histologic findings, and staining characteristics (see **Box 1**).
5. The development of detection assays optimized for cytologic samples will open the door to more widespread implementation of HPV testing, and may obviate tissue acquisition and processing.

REFERENCES

1. Gillison ML. Human papillomavirus-associated head and neck cancer is a distinct epidemiologic, clinical, and molecular entity. Semin Oncol 2004;31:744–54.
2. Gillison ML, Koch WM, Capone RB, et al. Evidence for a causal association between human papillomavirus and a subset of head and neck cancers. J Natl Cancer Inst 2000;92:709–20.
3. D'Souza G, Kreimer AR, Viscidi R, et al. Case-control study of human papillomavirus and oropharyngeal cancer. N Engl J Med 2007;356:1944–56.
4. Gillison ML, D'Souza G, Westra W, et al. Distinct risk factor profiles for human papillomavirus type 16-positive and human papillomavirus type 16-negative head and neck cancers. J Natl Cancer Inst 2008;100:407–20.
5. Begum S, Cao D, Gillison M, et al. Tissue distribution of human papillomavirus 16 DNA integration in patients with tonsillar carcinoma. Clin Cancer Res 2005;11: 5694–9.
6. El-Mofty SK, Zhang MQ, Davila RM. Histologic identification of human papillomavirus (HPV)-related squamous cell carcinoma in cervical lymph nodes: a reliable predictor of the site of an occult head and neck primary carcinoma. Head Neck Pathol 2008;2:163–8.
7. Westra WH. The changing face of head and neck cancer in the 21st century: the impact of HPV on the epidemiology and pathology of oral cancer. Head Neck Pathol 2009;3:78–81.
8. Ang KK, Harris J, Wheeler R, et al. Human papillomavirus and survival of patients with oropharyngeal cancer. N Engl J Med 2010;363:24–35.

9. Fakhry C, Westra WH, Li S, et al. Improved survival of patients with human papillomavirus-positive head and neck squamous cell carcinoma in a prospective clinical trial. J Natl Cancer Inst 2008;100:261–9.

10. Weinberger PM, Yu Z, Haffty BG, et al. Molecular classification identifies a subset of human papillomavirus-associated oropharyngeal cancers with favorable prognosis. J Clin Oncol 2006;24:736–47.

11. American Joint Committee on Cancer. AJCC cancer staging manual. New York: Springer; 2011.

12. Wenig BM, Barnes L, Carlson DL, et al. Protocol for the examination of specimens from patients with carcinomas of the pharynx. Northfield (MN): College of American Pathologists; 2011.

13. Singhi AD, Westra WH. Comparison of human papillomavirus in situ hybridization and p16 immunohistochemistry in the detection of human papillomavirus-associated head and neck cancer based on a prospective clinical experience. Cancer 2010;116:2166–73.

14. Begum S, Gillison ML, Ansari-Lari MA, et al. Detection of human papillomavirus in cervical lymph nodes: a highly effective strategy for localizing site of tumor origin. Clin Cancer Res 2003;9:6469–75.

15. Begum S, Gillison ML, Nicol TL, et al. Detection of human papillomavirus-16 in fine-needle aspirates to determine tumor origin in patients with metastatic squamous cell carcinoma of the head and neck. Clin Cancer Res 2007;13:1186–91.

16. Weichert W, Schewe C, Denkert C, et al. Molecular HPV typing as a diagnostic tool to discriminate primary from metastatic squamous cell carcinoma of the lung. Am J Surg Pathol 2009;33:513–20.

17. Cao D, Begum S, Ali SZ, et al. Expression of p16 in benign and malignant cystic squamous lesions of the neck. Hum Pathol 2010;41:535–9.

18. Zhao M, Rosenbaum E, Carvalho AL, et al. Feasibility of quantitative PCR-based saliva rinse screening of HPV for head and neck cancer. Int J Cancer 2005;117:605–10.

19. Worden FP, Kumar B, Lee JS, et al. Chemoselection as a strategy for organ preservation in advanced oropharynx cancer: response and survival positively associated with HPV16 copy number. J Clin Oncol 2008;26:3138–46.

20. Agrawal Y, Koch WM, Xiao W, et al. Oral human papillomavirus infection before and after treatment for human papillomavirus 16-positive and human papillomavirus 16-negative head and neck squamous cell carcinoma. Clin Cancer Res 2008;14:7143–50.

21. Chuang AY, Chuang TC, Chang S, et al. Presence of HPV DNA in convalescent salivary rinses is an adverse prognostic marker in head and neck squamous cell carcinoma. Oral Oncol 2008;44:915–9.

22. Paz IB, Cook N, Odom-Maryon T, et al. Human papillomavirus (HPV) in head and neck cancer. An association of HPV 16 with squamous cell carcinoma of Waldeyer's tonsillar ring. Cancer 1997;79:595–604.

23. Singhi AD, Califano J, Westra WH. High-risk human papillomavirus in nasopharyngeal carcinoma. Head Neck 2011;34(2):213–8.

24. Pai SI, Westra WH. Molecular pathology of head and neck cancer: implications for diagnosis, prognosis, and treatment. Annu Rev Pathol 2009;4:49–70.

25. El-Mofty SK, Lu DW. Prevalence of high-risk human papillomavirus DNA in nonkeratinizing (cylindrical cell) carcinoma of the sinonasal tract: a distinct clinicopathologic and molecular disease entity. Am J Surg Pathol 2005;29:1367–72.

26. Kim WY, Sharpless NE. The regulation of INK4/ARF in cancer and aging. Cell 2006;127:265–75.

27. Takeuchi S, Takahashi A, Motoi N, et al. Intrinsic cooperation between p16INK4a and p21Waf1/Cip1 in the onset of cellular senescence and tumor suppression in vivo. Cancer Res 2010;70:9381–90.
28. Strati K, Lambert PF. Role of Rb-dependent and Rb-independent functions of papillomavirus E7 oncogene in head and neck cancer. Cancer Res 2007;67: 11585–93.
29. Smeets SJ, Hesselink AT, Speel EJ, et al. A novel algorithm for reliable detection of human papillomavirus in paraffin embedded head and neck cancer specimen. Int J Cancer 2007;121:2465–72.
30. Robinson M, Sloan P, Shaw R. Refining the diagnosis of oropharyngeal squamous cell carcinoma using human papillomavirus testing. Oral Oncol 2010;46:492–6.
31. Hoffmann M, Ihloff AS, Gorogh T, et al. p16(INK4a) overexpression predicts translational active human papillomavirus infection in tonsillar cancer. Int J Cancer 2010;127:1595–602.
32. Klussmann JP, Gultekin E, Weissenborn SJ, et al. Expression of p16 protein identifies a distinct entity of tonsillar carcinomas associated with human papillomavirus. Am J Pathol 2003;162:747–53.
33. Shapiro GI, Park JE, Edwards CD, et al. Multiple mechanisms of p16INK4A inactivation in non-small cell lung cancer cell lines. Cancer Res 1995;55:6200–9.
34. Ukpo OC, Flanagan JJ, Ma XJ, et al. High-risk human papillomavirus E6/E7 mRNA detection by a novel in situ hybridization assay strongly correlates with p16 expression and patient outcomes in oropharyngeal squamous cell carcinoma. Am J Surg Pathol 2011;35:1343–50.
35. Jannapureddy S, Cohen C, Lau S, et al. Assessing for primary oropharyngeal or nasopharyngeal squamous cell carcinoma from fine needle aspiration of cervical lymph node metastases. Diagn Cytopathol 2010;38:795–800.
36. Umudum H, Rezanko T, Dag F, et al. Human papillomavirus genome detection by in situ hybridization in fine-needle aspirates of metastatic lesions from head and neck squamous cell carcinomas. Cancer 2005;105:171–7.
37. Zhang MQ, El-Mofty SK, Davila RM. Detection of human papillomavirus-related squamous cell carcinoma cytologically and by in situ hybridization in fine-needle aspiration biopsies of cervical metastasis: a tool for identifying the site of an occult head and neck primary. Cancer 2008;114:118–23.
38. Carozzi FM, Del Mistro A, Confortini M, et al. Reproducibility of HPV DNA testing by hybrid capture 2 in a screening setting. Am J Clin Pathol 2005;124:716–21.
39. IARC Working Group on the Evaluation of Cancer Preventive Strategies. Cervix cancer screening. Lyon (France): IARC Press; 2005.
40. Bishop JA, Maleki Z, Valsamakis A, et al. Application of the hybrid capture 2 assay to squamous cell carcinomas of the head and neck: a convenient liquid-phase approach for the reliable determination of human papillomavirus status. Cancer Cytopathol 2012;120(1):18–25.

Clinical Features of HPV-Related Head and Neck Squamous Cell Carcinoma: Presentation and Work-Up

Wayne M. Koch, MD

KEYWORDS

- Cystic nodal metastasis • Unknown primary • Palatine and lingual tonsils

KEY POINTS

- Human papillomavirus (HPV)-related head and neck squamous cell carcinoma (HNSCC) occurs predominantly in the lymphoepithelium of the oropharynx (OP): palatine and lingual tonsils (tongue base).
- Primary site of HPV-related HNSCC is difficult to detect, and in many instances cervical nodal metastases are the presenting sign of cancer (occult or unknown primary [UP] cancer).
- HPV-related HNSCC produces a distinct pattern of cystic cervical nodal metastasis.
- The risk profile for patients with HPV-related HNSCC is unlike that of traditional head and neck cancer, including individuals of early middle age who are nonsmokers or do not have an extensive tobacco history.
- Post-treatment surveillance of HPV-related HNSCC is affected by the improved response of this type of HNSCC to chemoradiation as well as a lower likelihood of second primary cancers arising in the upper aerodigestive tract (UADT).

INTRODUCTION

Squamous cell carcinoma (SCC) of the UADT associated with the presence of the HPV displays distinct clinical features that affect the presenting signs and symptoms of disease and can be used to help clinicians in diagnosis and work-up. These distinctive clinical features constitute powerful evidence for an active role of HPV in the etiology of HPV-related SCC.

SITE SPECIFICITY

One of the most specific and distinct features of HPV-related SCC is the region of the UADT in which it arises. HPV-related HNSCC arises predominantly in the

Disclosure: Nothing to disclose.
Department of Otolaryngology–Head and Neck Surgery, Johns Hopkins University School of Medicine, 601 North Caroline Street, Baltimore, MD 21287, USA
E-mail address: wkoch@jhmi.edu

Otolaryngol Clin N Am 45 (2012) 779–793
doi:10.1016/j.otc.2012.04.004
0030-6665/12/$ – see front matter © 2012 Elsevier Inc. All rights reserved.

oto.theclinics.com

lymphoepithelium of the OP in tissues commonly called tonsils. The tissue known as tonsils by the lay public is the palatine tonsils. The target of HPV-related tumorigenesis, however, includes both the palatine tonsils and the lingual tonsils. In a seminal article, Gillison and colleagues[1] showed that of 253 HNSCCs, all those with integrated HPV capable of tumor induction, were located in the OP, and oropharyngeal positive tumors arose predominantly from the palatine or lingual tonsils. Surface epithelial areas within the OP are not commonly associated with HPV-related SCC. Tumors of the uvula, soft palate, tonsillar pillars, and posterior pharyngeal wall do not typically contain HPV DNA. It may be difficult, however, to accurately identify the site of origin of large tumors that involve multiple subsites.

Controversy exists in the literature as to whether HPV-HNSCC arises in other sites within the UADT. Reports of a small number of laryngeal and oral cavity (OC) SCC lesions that contain HPV DNA appear occasionally. There may be several explanations for this:

1. HPV may truly affect mucosa outside the oropharyngeal lymphoepithelium under some undefined rare circumstances.
2. Laboratory methodology, such as polymerase chain reaction (PCR), used to identify HPV in some reports may have lower thresholds that result in categorizing a tumor as HPV positive when the amount of HPV signal is below biologic significance, indicative of laboratory background levels or simple infection without cancer transformation.
3. The true site of origin may be inaccurately recorded in the medical record. In the author's experience, this third explanation is often uncovered on closer examination of the medical record of cases with HPV-related tumor assigned to a non-OP site of origin. For example, the author found several cases in which samples taken from the oral tongue were found to be HPV-related HNSCC; however, the past history indicated that a tonsillectomy had been performed at an outside facility before the tongue biopsy was obtained and the tonsil specimen contained SCC. These cases are rightly categorized as having an OP primary site. The actual location of tissue taken from the vallecula or inferior lateral oropharyngeal wall may be called supraglottic larynx or hypopharynx, respectively, in cases where the epicenter of tumor is actually the tongue base or inferior palatine tonsil.

The reliance on surgical pathology reports alone to categorize the site of origin of a cancer case is problematic because specimens may be labeled in a manner that does not fully describe the orientation and extent of the entire tumor. Inexperience or lack of precision may lead a surgical endoscopist to mislabel the site from which a specimen is taken. Similarly, reports from computerized imaging may be misleading in that a radiologist is not always able to accurately locate a tumor boundary due to the contiguity and overlapping of structures in the UADT. The preponderance of a particular site of origin of HPV-related HNSCC in the OP in the majority of cases from virtually every report in the literature supports the author's contention that many if not all outlier cases could be explained by 1 of the 3 alternatives discussed previously.

One possible exception to this site specificity, which seems to be emerging, is the occasional presence of HPV-related SCC arising in the nasopharynx. Investigators at the University of Michigan reported that 4 cases of nasopharyngeal carcinoma in white subjects enrolled in a clinical trial had tumors that tested positive for HPV.[2] Recently, Singhi and colleagues[3] reported several cases in which nasopharyngeal biopsies were found to contain HPV whereas Epstein-Barr virus was more commonly associated with nasopharyngeal carcinoma. In all cases with available staging information, a tonsil lesion was also present.

The reason for the site specificity of HPV-related cancer to the tonsillar tissue of the OP is not fully understood. Lymphoepithelial tissue architecture seems designed to permit contact between external pathogens and the immune system. A permissively porous basement membrane has been described.[4] In addition, the deep crypts and irregularity of both the palatine and lingual tonsils may permit prolonged exposure of the epithelium with entrapped food debris and pathogens, which are protected from the purging of mucosal lining that regularly occurs elsewhere in the UADT with swallowing. There may be additional factors that link these physical features to explain the link between exposure, infection, and tumorigenesis.

OCCULT NATURE OF EARLY LESIONS

One clinically relevant effect of the origination of HPV-associated HNSCC in palatine and lingual tonsils is the occult nature of early lesions. Deep within tonsillar crypts or hidden amidst lingual tonsil fronds and mounds, early mucosal alterations due to HPV malignant transformation may grow undetected for many months. This is different than the early manifestation of cancers of the floor of mouth and ventral tongue in the OC. It is these OC tumors that are commonly associated with progression of leukoplakia and erythroplakia progressing from atypia to dysplasia. These OC lesions are also associated with field cancerization,[5] with multifocal tumors arising particularly in heavy smokers/drinkers. Field cancer effects are not seen in HPV-associated HNSCC, and precancer lesions in the tonsil and tongue base are rarely, if ever, reported. This is also different from the HPV-related precancer lesions seen on the uterine cervix and detected by Papanicolaou smear. The routine screening and accessibility of the cervical mucosa for testing of atypical cells and HPV DNA may facilitate early detection of precancerous changes—similar tests are not yet routinely available for OP screening.

OP tumors may grow to considerable size before causing symptoms, such as pain, dysphagia, or referred otalgia. Tonsillar asymmetry may be the presenting complaint, leading to a diagnosis of HPV-associated HNSCC. Finding a tumor in the tongue base is more difficult. The tongue base falls vertically away from the view of an examiner of the oral cavity, making it impossible to visualize without special equipment even for an interested examiner and a patient with a controlled gag reflex. When a laryngeal mirror or fiberoptic laryngoscope is used, the tongue base is still viewed tangentially, making thorough inspection difficult. Using a fiberoptic laryngoscope, examination is facilitated by maneuvers, such as asking the patient to protrude the tongue or puff the cheeks. The difficulty in visualizing and examining the tongue base and tonsil crypts contributes to a prolonged interval between presentation of an individual to a health care provider with complaints related to oropharyngeal cancer and the eventual diagnosis of the tumor. Although the interval between presentation and diagnosis is typically up to 9 months, there does not seem to be a negative impact on outcome of treatment attributable to this interval.[6]

Palpation of the tongue base is a vital part of the physical examination for early detection of base of tongue (BOT) tumors. Many care providers avoid BOT palpation fearing that a patient may vomit, bite, or refuse examination. The author finds that with proper preparation (explanation of the importance, encouragement to breathe steadily, and warning that patients will experience gag), BOT palpation is accepted and effective. This has been a standard part of the physical examination of the head and neck for many decades. What is being investigated is whether there are any discrete areas of increased firmness or raised mass effect in the tongue base. Examination in the clinic is limited not only by the gag reflex but also by tongue muscle turgor. A better evaluation is possible when patients are under general anesthesia with muscle relaxant in effect. Under these conditions, the extent of a tumor can be more easily assessed compared with the soft consistency of the tongue base musculature. Circumvallate papillae can feel firm and should not be mistaken for tumor. The size of these raised plaque-like taste organs is characteristically small (3 mm to 5 mm) and can be visualized while palpated to confirm their identity.

The site specificity of HPV-associated HNSCC is particularly relevant when searching for the primary tumor in cases where lymph node metastasis provides the initial histologic evidence of the cancer. If a node biopsy has confirmed HPV-associated cancer, the site of the primary tumor is very likely within the palatine or lingual tonsil. This is discussed in depth when UP cancer is considered.

NODAL DISEASE

The presenting sign of HPV-associated HNSCC frequently is the abrupt appearance of an enlarged cervical lymph node, which has implications in the diagnosis and evaluation of the disease. There are several other clinical details about HPV-associated HNSCC metastases that should be thoroughly understood. There are factors that contribute to the common phenomenon of a lymph node as the first and often only clinically apparent manifestation of HPV-associated HNSCC. First, the individuals affected often do not have the classical lifestyle risk exposures associated with HNSCC, specifically, extensive smoking and alcohol use, so are not considered at risk for the disease. Often people are not even aware that HNSCC exists before their own personal encounter. Another factor is the occult, symptom-free clinical course of many OP primary tumors. Many individuals who present with a metastatic lymph node enlargement report no problems related to the mouth or throat. It seems that HPV-associated oropharyngeal tumors often remain small in the face of large cervical metastases. Again, several factors may be at play: there may be a differential rate of tumor cell growth between primary and metastatic disease if the latter arises from a more transformed and more rapidly growing subclone of the tumor; metastatic tumor may have greater access to nutrients through proximity to blood vessels; and perhaps the predominant reason for the rapid appearance of large neck nodes in HPV-related HNSCC is the phenomenon of the cystic metastatic node.

For many years, the phenomenon of a cystic mass of recent onset presenting in the neck of young to middle-aged adults in whom SCC is found has been described. Reports in the literature of SCC arising in a branchial cleft cyst have been published and debated. The mechanism for malignant transformation of a benign epithelial cyst has been the subject of speculation. More recently, the observation that HPV-related SCC is often associated with cystic lymph node metastasis has been made.[7] A cystic lymph node is described as having a thin wall, containing clear liquid (**Fig. 1**). Because these nodes are often reported of recent abrupt onset, the mechanism for their growth may be obstruction and accumulation of lymphatic flow rather than growth of neoplastic cells beyond available blood supply with subsequent necrosis and liquification. In that case, the body of the mass is more irregular with areas of solid tumor and collections of caseous necrotic material.

The association of cystic nodal metastasis related to HPV-HNSCC is now so commonly recognized that the historical phenomenon of SCC arising in a branchial cleft cyst may be best reinterpreted as an early example of HPV-related disease. More importantly, any adult presenting with a new onset of a lateral cystic cervical mass should be suspected of having HPV-related HNSCC until proved otherwise. Lateral cystic neck masses appearing abruptly in adults should be worked up by fine-needle aspiration (FNA) with PCR of the aspirate looking for HPV DNA. If benign squamous epithelium is present, the most likely diagnosis remains metastatic SCC and further

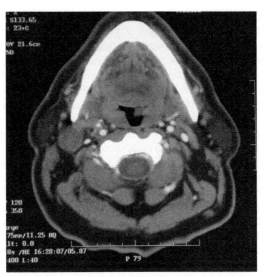

Fig. 1. Cystic cervical lymph node metastasis in HPV-related HNSCC.

work-up is warranted, including a direct laryngoscopy with directed biopsies. Ultrasound guidance may help identify areas of solid nodal metastases that coexist with a cystic node. If surgical extirpation is undertaken, the mass should be cleanly dissected, taking care not to violate the capsule, and the mass submitted for frozen histopathologic analysis. In anticipation of a cancer diagnosis, adequate operating room time should be requested and consent obtained for both completion neck dissection (at least regional, selective neck dissection) and examination under anesthesia with directed biopsies of the oropharyngeal lymphoepithelium in search of the primary tumor site. Failure to anticipate the likely diagnosis of cancer and to take these measures frequently results in suboptimal oncologic surgery with possible spillage of tumor cells and a need for revision surgery within a scarred field, putting vital structures, such as cranial nerves, at risk as well as losing an opportunity to complete the surgical diagnostic work-up under a single anesthetic.

A review of cystic cervical metastatic nodes at Johns Hopkins Hospital revealed that the majority of cases were from an HPV-related tonsil/tongue base primary.[7] Papillary thyroid carcinoma may also occasionally spawn cystic nodal metastasis. HPV-associated cystic nodes commonly occur, however, in the level II-III junction of the upper lateral neck to mid-lateral neck and achieve a larger size than papillary thyroid carcinoma cystic nodal metastases. Not all HPV-related SCC cervical nodal metastases are cystic; most are solid and commonly cystic and solid nodes coexist in the same patient.

Cystic metastasis may help explain two clinical phenomena: the abrupt appearance of large neck masses as a presenting sign of HPV-related HNSCC and an improved response rate to treatment of nodal metastasis in HPV-related HNSCCs compared with the formerly more common HNSCCs arising from exposure to tobacco and alcohol. In the first observation, rapid accumulation of lymphatic fluid may occur when a tumor implant reaches a size to block the effluent channels within a node. Fluid accumulation within a node may occur more quickly than would tumor parenchymal growth, consistent with the report of many patients that a node suddenly appeared and was noted, for example, while shaving. Similarly, if the substance of a nodal metastasis is largely lymphatic fluid, the size on which nodal staging is based is inflated and disproportionate to the actual tumor burden. There are orders of magnitude fewer viable tumor cells in an 8 cm³ (2 × 2 × 2 cm) cystic node compared with a solid nodal metastasis of the same size. The responsiveness of HPV-related HNSCC to various treatments seems better than that of non-HPV–related cancer, ostensibly because of a less disrupted genetic milieu in tumors that undergo malignant transformation because of the effect of the E6 and E7 HPV oncoproteins. Stage inflation, however, in which nodal metastases with small tumor volumes are graded as N2 or N3 disease, may also contribute to an apparent improvement in clinical outcome. This phenomenon may have a role in the current debate about the necessity for a "planned" neck dissection in which a neck dissection is done after treatment regardless of clinical response when the presenting disease stage is N2 or above. This dogma may be less warrented for HPV-related HNSCC.

The position of cervical nodal metastasis from HPV-related HNSCC primary disease is also highly characteristic. As discussed previously, the deep jugular nodal chain in the upper-mid neck is the typical location for these metastases. Nodal disease that appears more anteriorly, even along the common facial vein between levels I and II, is suggestive of a non-HPV–related source. Both the palatine and lingual tonsils can spawn contralateral nodal metastases. In most cases, this is in conjunction with ipsilateral metastases but can occur as an isolated event, which is important in informing the strategy of looking for an occult primary tumor as well as in design of the scope of neck treatment (radiation or surgery) required in these cases. Another consideration is the propensity for nodal metastasis from the palatine tonsil to spread to retropharyngeal nodes. These lymph nodes are difficult to approach surgically and are not typically removed at the time of a comprehensive nodal dissection. Again, the potential for nodal metastasis to an area behind the posterior pharyngeal wall may be indication to include the tonsil region in radiation portals even when a tonsil primary tumor has been completely resected.

WORK-UP OF HPV-RELATED HNSCC

Work-up for cancer begins with the presentation of a patient with a clinical picture that raises the possibility of cancer in the differential diagnosis (**Table 1**). The likelihood of entertaining a possible cancer diagnosis is based on an index of suspicion and is a form of profiling that calls on the knowledge and experience of clinicians to narrow the spectrum of possibility to a diagnosis considered plausible or likely.

- The phenomenon of HPV-related HNSCC has dramatically changed the expected profile of HNSCC patients from that of mostly 45-year-old to 75-year-old men with an extensive history of smoking and drinking to a much wider group of otherwise healthy slightly younger (35–55 years) individuals, still mostly men but less likely to have a significant tobacco history.
- A history of multiple sexual partners, in particular orogenital partners, is evidenced by careful epidemiologic studies as a risk factor,[8] but this history is more sensitive and less commonly obtained than is information about tobacco and alcohol use.
- The possibility that marijuana use is also a contributing factor to HPV-associated HNSCC development has been raised,[8] again adding a new and sensitive component to the social history that could lead to an appropriate elevation of index of suspicion.
- There is also some suggestion in the literature that HPV-related HNSCC is disproportionately common in whites, although more data are needed to corroborate this observation.[9]

Table 1
Work-up of HPV-related head and neck squamous cell carcinoma

History	
Presenting sign/symptoms	Neck mass (abrupt appearance); chronic sore throat; referred otalgia; asymptomatic
Risk profile	Nonsmokers > smokers; male > female; white > black; multiple oral sex partners
Physical Examination	
Primary site	Inspection, including fiberoptic pharyngoscopy; palpation of palatine tonsils and tongue base
Neck	Size, mobility, firmness, and region (level II–IV bilateral)
Radiography	CT with intravenous contrast Cystic nodal metastasis MRI, PET, ultrasound
Biopsy	
Clinic	FNA of lymph node; accessible tonsil/BOT with local anesthesia
Operating room	Examination under anesthesia with palpation Tonsillectomy (bilateral) Biopsy of tongue base directed visually and by palpation
Pathology	HPV testing (HPV quantitative PCR/in situ hybridization)

The result of this shift in risk profile is that it is appropriate to consider HPV-related HNSCC in the differential diagnosis of individuals presenting with other fairly common findings (neck mass, persistent sore throat, and tonsil hypertrophy) in a wide range of individuals. Although HPV-related HNSCC is still an uncommon disease (approximately 20,000 cases per year in the US population), it must be considered a possible diagnosis more readily than in the past. Compared with oral cancer, which the dental community has increasingly begun regular screening to detect, HPV-related HNSCC is more common and less immediately visible on simple inspection.

Although the range of presenting signs and symptoms for HPV-related HNSCC is broad, several features stand out.

- The primary tumor site may cause no symptoms and may remain hidden for an extended period of time, resulting in diagnosis after metastasis to a cervical lymph node with the presentation of a new neck mass.
- Persistent nodal hypertrophy (more than 2 cm in greatest dimension) not responding to medical therapy and remaining unchanged for 4 to 6 weeks should invoke the possibility of HPV-associated HNSCC, particularly when the node is in the upper jugular chain. These nodes are typically firm, discrete, mobile, and nontender.
- Alternatively, a persistent sore throat localized to the OP with or without referred otalgia should raise the consideration of tonsil and tongue base disease. Again, initial medical therapy, including antibiotics or gastroesophageal reflux medication, may be undertaken but, if not effective in 4 to 6 weeks, the clinician should give way to alternatives in the differential diagnosis, including HPV-related HNSCC.
- Visible asymmetry of the tonsils, difficulty with swallowing, pharyngeal bleeding, and change in voice are less common and suggest more advanced disease.

PHYSICAL EXAMINATION

Visual inspection of the palatine tonsils using a flashlight and tongue depressor is possible in most individuals. In some cases, even this maneuver invokes an immediate and strong gag reflex, rendering an adequate view unobtainable. Fiberoptic nasopharyngoscopy is useful for the tongue base but does not help with assessment of the palatine tonsils. Even when the primary cancer is in the palatine tonsil, it is visible only after there is sufficient tumor volume to result in tonsil asymmetry because often the overlying surface mucosa is uninvolved with tumor.

- A tag of friable papillomatous tissue, areas of discoloration, and/or bleeding are rare signs of tonsil cancer.
- Similarly, unilateral mass tonsil hypertrophy is uncommonly caused by HPV-associated HNSCC. Healthy tonsils may appear asymmetric due to the position of the lymphoepithelial tissue within the tonsil fossa, with one tonsil more protrusive from the anterior and posterior pillar whereas another is more deeply inset. The actual comparability in tonsil volume in these cases may be demonstrated by CT scan.
- True asymmetry or bilateral tonsillar hypertrophy may also be indicative of lymphoma (mucosa-associated lymphoid tissue), which should be included in the differential diagnosis along with HPV-related HNSCC.

Examination of Tonsil

Palpation of the palatine tonsil is tolerated by some patients, and, if so, may allow the clinician to locate small areas of induration or overall increase in turgor in an affected tonsil. For patients with significant active gag reflex, this careful palpation may best be performed under general anesthesia at the time of direct laryngoscopy.

Examination of Tongue Base

The tongue base is even more challenging to examine than is the palatine tonsil. In a few individuals, the tongue base may be visible on simple oral inspection; in a few people, even the epiglottis is visible with the help of a flashlight. The lingual tonsils, however, are located on a vertically oriented surface, blocked from view by the oral tongue and further obscured by a normal gag reflex. The use of a laryngeal mirror or fiberoptic nasopharyngoscopy is usually required to view the lingual tonsil surface. Because of the nodular surface of the normal tongue base, all but the most obvious and large tumors are not easily detected by visual inspection. Areas of slight color alteration (red, purple, or white), subtle restriction of motion with tongue protrusion or swallowing, or slight increase in contour or irregularity of nodularity compared with the lingual tonsil mounds may be detected. Again, palpation can be of immense help in some cases. The characteristic firmness of an indurated tumor growth becomes familiar with experience and serves to confirm suspicion.

Examination of Neck

The examination of the neck for lymph node metastasis is also a skill that must be developed. Comparison of the right and left nodal basins is facilitated by standing behind a patient during the examination and using the tips of the index and third finger to palpate tissues while rolling the sternocleidomastoid muscle backward. Up-and-down or side-to-side motion provides information about the size, mobility, consistency, demarcation of periphery, and number of nodes. The body habitus plays a role in the effectiveness of the neck examination; heavy, short-necked, and muscular individuals are more difficult to examine. Particular attention is given to both jugular chains when HPV-related HNSCC is suspected. Two centimeters is a useful starting point for concern about a node. The width of an index finger of most adult clinicians is approximately 1.5 cm to 2 cm. Smaller nodes that are round and unusually firm may also warrant attention, particularly when accompanying a more obvious patho-logically enlarged node.

RADIOGRAPHY

Radiographic imaging is commonly undertaken when the history and physical exam-ination suggest HNSCC.

CT and MRI

CT and MRI are both useful for evaluation of the primary site in tonsil and tongue base as well as the nodal basin. When CT is done, intravenous contrast is invaluable to distinguish nodes from vessels and to provide evidence of neovascular blush in the tumor primary (**Fig. 2**B). MRI scans are particularly helpful to discern the extent of tongue base involvement in many HNSCC cases (see **Fig. 2**C), although the contact between surfaces within the resting OP may be misinterpreted as tumor involvement in adjacent structures. Computerized imaging also informs tumor staging by providing precise measurements of primary and metastatic masses.

PET

Positron emission tomography (PET) scanning is increasingly available; although, because of its high cost, its use is often restricted to cases already having a cancer diagnosis (see **Fig. 2**A). Although uptake of radiolabeled glucose is strongly associ-ated with malignant growth, it also may be present during inflammation. For that reason, the sites of oropharyngeal biopsies may demonstrate PET positive uptake for several weeks during the healing process. Even normal palatine and lingual tonsils demonstrate some degree of PET uptake due to chronic inflammation inherent in these structures. PET scans superimposed on CT images taken at the same setting are preferable to identify the active structure with a higher degree of certainty (**Fig. 3**).

Ultrasound

Ultrasound is helpful for examination of the lateral neck nodal basins but has not been used to detect the character of the tonsillar tissues. As in other malignant metastatic conditions, ultrasonography provides precise size measurements of involved nodes as well as documenting the loss of normal architecture (oval shape and fatty hilum)

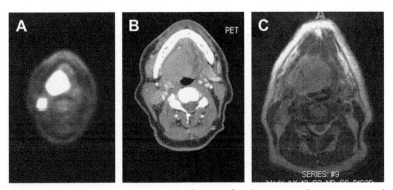

Fig. 2. (*A*) PET, (*B*) CT with contrast, and (*C*) MRI of right tongue base tumor and nodal metastasis.

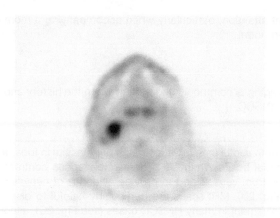

Fig. 3. PET scan of right neck SCC in neck node with UP. Note low level of fluorodeoxyglucose uptake in lingual tonsil tissue bilaterally, which is physiologic.

and the presence of increased vascular supply. Although ultrasound may have a role for the evaluation of cervical lymphadenopathy, it does not replace CT or MRI scanning to assess lymph node involvement in relation to other structures in the neck.

BIOPSY AND EXAMINATION UNDER ANESTHESIA

No diagnosis of cancer can be made without a confirmatory biopsy. Obtaining tumor tissue for rigorous HPV testing (in situ hybridization or quantitative PCR) is the only way to confirm that HNSCC is HPV related. Although some clinicians and patients may be able to cooperate sufficiently in an office to allow an adequate biopsy of the palatine or even the lingual tonsils, general anesthesia is required in most cases and facilitates the thorough assessment needed to appropriately stage and document the extent of disease.

Palatine Tonsils

In an operating room, the palatine tonsils can be visualized fully using a tonsil gag to open the mouth and depress the tongue. Adequate biopsy may require a complete tonsillectomy, removing the palatine tonsil from the tonsil fossa. For the occult primary tumors, bilateral tonsillectomy is warranted to localize small tumors, which may not be palpable and amenable to directed biopsies.[10,11] For large palpable tumors, cup forceps or other instruments can be used to harvest pieces of tumor for histologic evaluation.

Tongue Base

Again, the tongue base provides a greater challenge than does the tonsil arch even in the setting of general anesthesia.

Palpation

Palpation with a gloved finger before any laryngoscopic examination can be useful. With the tongue musculature relaxed, the increased turgor of tumor is more readily recognized, and the precise limits of the tumor can be discerned. Surgeons should pay particular attention to involvement beyond midline, to the availability of adequate normal tongue base on one side or another to protect a neurovascular pedicle should surgery be undertaken, and to the involvement of the vallecula at the level of the hyoid bone. The latter is indicative of an ability to remove tumor without requiring removal of the epiglottis, which is critical to avoiding aspiration if the larynx is left intact. All these features are best determined by palpation rather than instrumentation.

Rigid endoscopy

Because of the location, surface contour, and orientation of the tongue base, the use of a rigid laryngoscope is necessary to inspect the lingual tonsils. Illuminated rigid endoscopy is performed after palpation to evaluate the soft, deformable tongue base for subtle signs of color change and friability. Palpation with a rigid suction can provide information about tumor induration. If tumor is visible, its extent with respect to the midline, the epiglottis, lateral pharyngeal walls, and oral tongue beyond the circumvallate papillae is noted. Tongue base biopsy sites are selected by identification of visible tumor but also may be directed by the palpating finger if the tumor can be reached by palpation. An upbiting cup forceps designed for laryngoscopy can be directed along the palpating finger until the jaws are at the fingertip and then pushed forward to engage the palpable tumor.

PANENDOSCOPY

The standard practice of including esophagoscopy and bronchoscopy in the work-up of HNSCC is challenged by the phenomenon of HPV-associated HNSCC. HPV-associated disease, unlike that produced by tobacco exposure, is rarely multifocal due to the absence of a field cancerization effect. Although 5% to 10% of all cases of HNSCC arising in heavy smokers may coexist with a metachronous second primary elsewhere in the UADT, the majority of HPV-related cases involve only one primary site. Furthermore, the advent of PET scanning alters the rationale for panendoscopy by augmenting the scope of radiographic imaging to permit detection of small mucosal primaries in the esophagus and tracheobronchial tree.

STAGING

Tumor stage for HNSCC in the OP is straightforward. The primary tumor stage (T) is based on the greatest diameter of the tumor, with special account taken for extension beyond the OP and deep tissue invasion in advanced stages. The nodal stage (N) is also based on the size of the lymph node metastasis as well as the site relative to the primary tumor and the number of nodes with metastatic implants. Although extranodal extension (extracapsular spread) of tumor outside a lymph node is of profound prognostic significance, it is not incorporated into the existing staging schema. The overall stage (I–IV) is then based on a formula combining the T and N stages (**Box 1**).

UNKNOWN PRIMARY

HNSCC that presents as lymph node metastasis but in which no primary site is detected is termed HNSCC of UP. When the literature on UP is evaluated, it must first be noted as to the point in the work-up at which the designation has been applied.

- Has an expert in head and neck cancer examined the patient?
- Have high-quality imaging studies been obtained?
- Has an examination under anesthesia with biopsies been performed?

Box 1
Staging of oropharyngeal SCC

Primary tumor (T)

- TX: primary tumor cannot be assessed
- T0: no evidence of primary tumor
- Tis: carcinoma in situ
- T1: tumor ≤2 cm in greatest dimension
- T2: tumor >2 cm but ≤4 cm in greatest dimension
- T3: tumor >4 cm in greatest dimension
- T4a: tumor invades adjacent structures (medial pterygoid muscle/s, mandible, hard palate, deep muscle of tongue, larynx)
- T4b: tumor invades lateral pterygoid muscle, pterygoid plates, lateral nasopharynx, or skull base or encases carotid artery

Nodal metastasis (N)

- N1: single lymph node metastasis, ipsilateral to primary tumor, <3 cm diameter
- N2a: single lymph node metastasis, ipsilateral to primary tumor, >3 cm and <6 cm diameter
- N2b: multiple lymph node metastases, all ipsilateral to primary tumor, all <6 cm diameter
- N2c: lymph node metastasis contralateral to primary tumor, with or without coexisting ipsilateral nodes, all <6 cm in diameter
- N3: Lymph node metastasis >6 cm in diameter

Stage grouping

- I: T1N0
- II: T2N0
- III: T3N0, T1N1, T2N1, T3N1
- IVA: T4aN0, T4aN1, any TN2
- IVB: T4b any N, any TN3
- IVC: Any T, any N, M1

From AJCC staging manual. 6th edition. New York: Springer-Verlag; 2003. p. 47–60; with permission.

This discussion begins with a patient in whom a lymph node with SCC has been documented but no symptoms or visible signs of cancer primary site are detected. If the nodal metastasis is cystic or if an FNA has been adequate for HPV or p16 testing, the OP is appropriately the focus of the initial search for the primary site.

An expert clinician begins with a focused history and thorough physical examination, including palpation of the palatine and lingual tonsils. Thorough fiberoptic evaluation of the tongue base is performed. CT scan with intravenous contrast or MRI is obtained and evaluated by a cancer specialist, not just by a radiologist. PET scans may be obtained at this point, given the confirmation of cancer by node FNA. The increased sensitivity of PET scans for malignant growth is partially offset by a lack of specificity, particularly in the lymphoepithelium (see **Fig. 3**). The efficacy of PET scanning to identify an UP in the UADT remains a subject of debate.[12,13]

Examination under anesthesia is the next step in work-up of the UP. Palpation and visual inspection are followed by complete bilateral tonsillectomy if patients have not had previous tonsil removal. The removal of all palatine tonsil tissue increases the likelihood of a pathologist identifying a primary site even when small and in the depth of the tonsil crypts.[10] The author sends the ipsilateral tonsil for inspection in the pathology laboratory and for frozen section analysis. If a primary tumor is discovered, further biopsies are not needed. The removal of the contralateral tonsil provides 2 advantages:

1. It removes a second possible primary site because some palatine tonsil cancers spawn contralateral nodal metastasis.[11]
2. It removes tissue that would otherwise continue to show glucose uptake on follow-up surveillance PET scanning, raising questions about the possible presence of second primary disease.

If the ipsilateral tonsil does not contain the primary site, extensive tongue base tissue sampling is performed, particularly on the ipsilateral side but including the entire tongue base. Several groups have begun to employ a robot to assist in comprehensive lingual tonsillectomy in selected cases. Only if all of these measures fail to identify a primary tumor site is the case truly one of UP and appropriately considered subject to full radiation of all the Waldeyer ring.

POST-TREATMENT SURVEILLANCE

After radiation-based treatment of HPV-related HNSCC, surveillance to ensure the prolonged absence of disease is critical. Precise documentation of the original extent of disease is important to direct attention of the examiner. Nonsmokers with HPV-related disease are not subject to second primary cancer development to an extent comparable with that of smokers with field cancerization at play. Still, the challenges of examining the OP, in particular the tongue base, remain after treatment. Patients seem more resigned and perhaps less sensitive to the palpating finger examination that is a key component of surveillance visits, as it was during initial work-up. The drying and thickening of tissues changes visual and tactile features of the tonsil and tongue base. Persistent pain is a particularly worrisome sign and warrants examination under anesthesia and repeat biopsy in most cases.

SUMMARY

1. HPV-related HNSCC is primarily a disease of the lymphoepithelium of the oropharynx. Reports of HPV in SCC arising in the OC and larynx are common but may be misleading. With careful review of individual case records, many of these cases can be demonstrated to have arisen from the OP and have been misclassified because of subsequent biopsy of persistent disease in an adjacent site or because of extension of disease to an adjacent site. In other reports, PCR evidence alone is offered to indicate that a tumor is HPV related. Rigorous methods, such as quantitative PCR, in situ hybridization, and Southern blotting, indicate that HPV is present in amounts adequate to be present in all tumor cells and, therefore, to be biologically active in malignant transformation only in OP cases. The reasons for this site specificity are not fully understood. The nasopharynx is a possible exception to this assertion of OP site specificity with recent reports of isolated cases of nasopharyngeal disease containing HPV DNA. Whether these are cases in which tonsillar lymphoepithelial rests are located above the soft palate or whether HPV has affected the nasopharyngeal epithelium directly remains to be ascertained.
2. Bilateral tonsillectomy should be performed when searching for an HPV-related primary site in individuals who have not had a prior tonsillectomy. Although

ipsilateral tonsillectomy may be sufficient to identify an occult primary in a majority of cases, there have been reports of contralateral spread of disease and a few reports of small sites of cancer in both tonsils. More importantly, removal of the uninvolved tonsil simplifies post-treatment surveillance by eliminating the uptake in the normal remaining tonsil that may be misinterpreted as suspicious for recurrent or second primary disease.

3. PET scans should be performed in the work-up of all cases of HPV-related HNSCC. Although PET may not be useful in identifying an occult primary site in all cases, it is helpful in examination of the retropharyngeal nodal basin and the contralateral neck. Improvements in PET scanning take into account the background activity of lymphoepithelial mucosa, which could enhance the specificity in identifying small primary tumors.

4. Panendoscopy is not needed in cases of HPV-related HNSCC. Traditional teaching regarding the work-up of HNSCC indicates the need to perform esophagoscopy and bronchoscopy because of a 5% to 10% risk of a second primary cancer presenting at the time of work-up. This is true among individuals with extensive tobacco and alcohol exposure history, but among HPV-related cancer patients, the rate of second UADT primary cancer seems much lower. Long-term follow-up studies of large cohorts of HPV-related HNSCC cancer patients are needed to confirm the distinctive absence of risk of second primary UADT cancer in this population. Post-treatment surveillance schedules may then be tailored to this population.

5. The concept of SCC arising in a branchial cleft cyst has been discredited. Such cases represent cystic nodal metastases from an HPV-related HNSCC. Any adult presenting with a new onset of a lateral neck cyst should undergo FNA before excision. If there are squamous cells present in the aspirate, even if of benign cytology, the surgical approach should include preparation for completion neck dissection and examination under anesthesia with biopsy to identify the primary site.

6. Thorough palpation of the tongue base is an essential part of the office evaluation of patients during work-up for possible HPV-related HNSCC. Although some clinicians assert that this cannot be performed because of the danger of patients gagging with vomiting, it is well tolerated by properly prepared patients who understand its importance and are aware that brief gagging sensation is expected. Palpation of the tongue base is more effective in identifying small suspicious areas of primary tumor than is visualization in many instances.

REFERENCES

1. Gillison ML, Koch WM, Capone RB, et al. Evidence for a causal association between human papillomavirus and a subset of head and neck cancers. J Natl Cancer Inst 2000;92(9):709–20.

2. Maxwell JH, Kumar B, Feng FY, et al. Bradford CR. HPV-positive/p16-positive/EBV-negative nasopharyngeal carcinoma in white North Americans. Head Neck 2010;32(5):562–7.

3. Singhi AD, Califano J, Westra WH. High-risk human papillomavirus in nasopharyngeal carcinoma. Head Neck 2012;34(2):213–8.

4. Westra WH. The changing face of head and neck cancer in the 21st century: the impact of HPV on the epidemiology and pathology of oral cancer. Head Neck Pathol 2009;3(1):78–81.

5. Slaughter DP, Southwick HW, Smejkal W. Field cancerization in oral stratified squamous epithelium; clinical implications of multicentric origin. Cancer 1953; 6(5):963–8.

6. Ho T, Zahurek M, Koch WM. Prognostic significance of presentation-to-diagnosis interval in patients with oropharyngeal carcinoma. Arch Otolaryngol Head Neck Surg 2004;130:45–51.

7. Goldenberg D, Begum S, Westra WH, et al. Cystic lymph node metastasis in patients with head and neck cancer: an HPV-associated phenomenon. Head Neck 2008;30(7):898–903.

8. D'Souza G, Kreimer AR, Viscidi R, et al. Case-control study of human papillomavirus and oropharyngeal cancer. N Engl J Med 2007;356(19):1944–56.

9. Schrank TP, Han Y, Weiss H, et al. Case-matching analysis of head and neck squamous cell carcinoma in racial and ethnic minorities in the United States— possible role for human papillomavirus in survival disparities. Head Neck 2011; 33(1):45–53.

10. McQuone SJ, Eisele DW, Lee DJ, et al. Occult tonsillar carcinoma in the unknown primary. Laryngoscope 1998;108:1605–10.

11. Koch WM, Bhatti N, Williams MF, et al. Oncologic rationale for bilateral tonsillectomy for head and neck squamous cell carcinoma of an unknown primary source. Otolaryngol Head Neck Surg 2001;124:331–3.

12. Wartski M, Le Stanc E, Gontier E, et al. In search of an unknown primary tumour presenting with cervical metastases: performance of hybrid FDG-PET-CT. Nucl Med Commun 2007;28(5):365–71.

13. Silva P, Hulse P, Sykes AJ, et al. Should FDG-PET scanning be routinely used for patients with an unknown head and neck squamous primary? J Laryngol Otol 2007;121(2):149–53.

Impact of HPV-Related Head and Neck Cancer in Clinical Trials
Opportunity to Translate Scientific Insight into Personalized Care

Christine H. Chung, MD[a],*, David L. Schwartz, MD[b,c,d]

KEYWORDS

- Human papillomavirus • Head and neck cancer • Chemotherapy • Radiotherapy
- Clinical trials • Biomarkers

KEY POINTS

- Patients with human papillomavirus (HPV)-positive squamous cell carcinoma of the oropharynx (SCCOP) have favorable clinical outcomes relative to patients with HPV-negative SCCOP.
- Patient selection with validated biomarkers is critical for personalized clinical trial design.
- HPV-associated SCCOP represents an opportunity for careful treatment deintensification to reduce toxicity. New radiotherapy, less invasive surgery, and systemic treatment options serve to make this a feasible goal.
- New approaches are required to identify and treat HPV-negative SCCOP at the highest risk for treatment failure.

INTRODUCTION

Squamous cell carcinoma of the head and neck (SCCHN) is a heterogeneous disease arising from various subsites within the head and neck region. As cigarette use has declined over the past 3 decades in the United States, there has been a gratifying reduction in the incidence of oral cavity, larynx, and hypopharynx cancers.[1] In stark contrast, the incidence of SCCOP has been steadily increasing,[2] and the literature demonstrates that

Funding support: None.
Conflict of interest: None.
[a] Department of Oncology, Johns Hopkins University School of Medicine, 1650 Orleans Street, CRB-1 Room 344, Baltimore, MD 21231-1000, USA; [b] Department of Radiation Medicine, Hofstra North Shore LIJ School of Medicine, 270-05 76th Avenue, New Hyde Park, NY 11040, USA; [c] Department of Otolaryngology, Hofstra North Shore LIJ School of Medicine, 270-05 76th Avenue, New Hyde Park, NY 11040, USA; [d] Department of Molecular Medicine, Hofstra North Shore LIJ School of Medicine, 270-05 76th Avenue, New Hyde Park, NY 11040, USA
* Corresponding author.
E-mail address: Cchung11@JHMI.Edu

the common etiologic factor for this new population of patients is pharyngeal infection with oncogenic strains of HPV.[3,4] The epidemiologic and pathophysiologic differences between HPV-positive SCCOP and HPV-negative SCCOP, as well as methods of HPV detection, are discussed in the articles by Fakhry, Westra and Pai elsewhere in this issue. This article focuses on the impact of HPV infection in clinical trials and patient care.

The ultimate goal of therapeutic clinical trials is to develop novel, safe, and efficacious therapies for patients that can improve clinical outcomes. To bring experimental agents from laboratories to clinics, they have to undergo multiple testing steps through preclinical studies and phase I, II, and III clinical trials. Once safety and efficacy are established in phase I and II trials, randomized phase III clinical trials are conducted for a comparison with the current standard of care. To avoid bias in the treatment arms and allow comparisons from trials to trials, clearly defining the study population through strict eligibility criteria is important. Traditionally the eligibility criteria included general clinical parameters, such as age, tumor histology, disease stage, performance status, and hematological and nonhematological end-organ function measures. It has been known, however, that these clinical parameters include heterogeneous patient populations with various outcomes given the same treatment. With these limitations in patient selection, various biomarkers were developed in an attempt to further molecularly define the disease with information gained from laboratory studies in addition to existing clinical parameters. One of the most powerful prognostic biomarkers found to date is HPV status in SCCHN.

Retrospective identification of improved treatment response and control of HPV-positive tumors in completed phase II trials is summarized in **Table 1**.[5–7] One of the first studies showing this prognostic difference was a secondary analysis of the Eastern Cooperative Oncology Group (ECOG) phase II clinical trial E2399. This study was originally designed to determine the role of induction chemotherapy followed by concurrent chemoradiotherapy for organ preservation in resectable stage III or IV squamous cell carcinoma of the larynx or oropharynx.[8] Patients with HPV-positive tumors had significantly higher response rate and longer progression-free survival (PFS) and overall survival (OS).[5] In a multivariate analysis adjusting for age, tumor stage, ECOG performance status, and tumor HPV status, HPV status was an independent prognostic variable.

With the preliminary but powerful evidence that the HPV status may have a significant impact in patient care and outcome, secondary post hoc analyses of tumor samples from several phase III clinical trials have been conducted (**Table 2**).[9–14] The first study to confirm these findings was from the phase III Radiation Therapy Oncology Group (RTOG) 0129 trial.[9] This trial was originally designed to compare standard-fractionation radiotherapy and cisplatin with accelerated-fractionation radiotherapy and cisplatin. Of the 721 patients enrolled, 323 (45%) patients had the oropharyngeal primary subsite with available tissue samples for HPV testing. Among these patients, 206 of 323 (64%) were HPV positive according to in situ hybridization and 214 of 323 (66%) were positive for p16 protein overexpression by immunohistochemistry as a surrogate marker of biologically active HPV infection. Consistent with the earlier studies, the demographics of patients with HPV-positive tumors were distinct from the patients with HPV-negative tumors. These patients were of younger age, had less-extensive tobacco exposure histories, and enjoyed better performance status. Furthermore, the patients with HPV-positive tumors had smaller primary tumors and more-extensive lymph node metastasis relative to patients with HPV-negative tumors. Although the clinical outcomes between the 2 comparison arms were not significantly different, secondary analysis confirmed significantly superior survival in patients with HPV-positive tumors versus HPV-negative disease.

Table 1
Retrospective analyses of HPV status and survival outcomes in phase II clinical trials

Study	Subsite	Treatment Regimen	HPV Status			Progression-Free Survival			Overall Survival		
			N (n)	Pos (%)	Neg (%)	HPV+	HPV−	Log Rank (P Value)	HPV+	HPV−	Log Rank (P Value)
E2399 Fakhry et al[5]	L or OP	Sequential therapy: paclitaxel/carboplatin radiation 70 Gy + paclitaxel	105 (96)	38 (40)	58 (60)	2-y (86%)	2-y (53%)	0.02	2-y (95%)	2-y (62%)	0.005
UMCC 9921 Worden et al[6]	OC, OP, HP, or L	Sequential therapy: cisplatin/5-fluorouracil or carboplatin/ 5-fluorouracil Responders: radiation + cisplatin or Nonresponders: surgery + radiation	66 (42)	27 (64)	15 (36)	Favorable prognosis for HPV+ (P = .004)			Favorable prognosis for HPV+ (P = .008)		
Kies et al[7]	OC, OP, HP, L, or NP	Sequential therapy: carboplatin/paclitaxel/ cetuximab Early stage: radiation 66–72 Gy or Late stage: 66–72 Gy + cisplatin or carboplatin	47 (26)	12 (46)	14 (54)	Favorable prognosis for HPV+ (P = .012)			Favorable prognosis for HPV+ (P = .046)		

Abbreviations: HP, hypopharynx; L, larynx; n, number of patients tested for HPV status; N, total number of patients enrolled; Neg, negative; NP, nasopharynx; OC, oral cavity; OP, oropharynx; Pos, positive.

Table 2
Retrospective analyses of HPV status and/or p16 immunohistochemical staining status as a surrogate biomarker of HPV infection and survival outcomes in phase III clinical trials

Study	Subsite	Treatment Regimen	N (n)	HPV or p16 Status		Progression-Free Survival			Overall Survival		
				Pos (%)	Neg (%)	HPV+/p16+	HPV−/p16−	Log Rank (P Value)	HPV+/p16+	HPV−/p16−	Log-Rank (P Value)
RTOG 0129 Ang et al[9]	OC, OP, HP, or L	Standard-fractionated radiation + cisplatin vs hyperfractionated radiation + cisplatin (no survival differences seen between the 2 treatment arms)	743 (323)	HPV: 206 (64) p16: 215 (68)	HPV: 117 (36) p16: 101 (32)	3-y HPV (74%) 3-y p16 (74%)	3-y HPV (43%) 3-y p16 (38%)	HPV <0.001 p16 <0.001	3-y HPV (82%) 3-y p16 (84%)	3-y HPV (57%) 3-y p16 (51%)	HPV <0.001 p16 <0.001
DAHANCA 5 Lassen et al[10,11]	OP, HP, NP, or L	Radiation vs Radiation + nimorazole	195 (156) 219 (175)	p16: 35 (22) p16: 49 (28)	p16: 121 (78) p16: 126 (72)	5-y^a p16 (70%)	5-y^a p16 (40%)	NA	5-y p16 (62%)	5-y p16 (26%)	0.0003
DAHANCA 6&7 Lassen et al[12]	OC, OP, HP, NP, or L	5 Fractions/wk radiation vs 6 Fractions/wk radiation	726 (385) 750 (409)	p16: 84 (22) p16: 95 (23)	p16: 301 (78) p16: 314 (77)	5-y^a p16 (78%)	5-y^a p16 (64%)	p16 0.001	5-y p16 (62%)	5-y p16 (47%)	<0.0001
TROG 02.02 Rischin et al[13]	OC, OP, HP, or L	Radiation + cisplatin vs radiation + cisplatin + tirapazamine (no survival differences seen between the 2 treatment arms)	861 (185)	p16: 106 (57)	p16: 79 (43)	2-y^b p16 (87%)	2-y^b p16 (72%)	p16 0.003	2-y p16 (91%)	2-y p16 (74%)	0.004

| TAX 324 Posner et al[14] | OC, OP, HP, or L | Induction chemotherapy regimen Docetaxel/cisplatin/5-fluorouracil vs cisplatin/5-fluorouracil (no survival differences seen between the 2 treatment arms in the subset of HPV-tested patients) | 501 (111) | HPV: 56 (50) | HPV: 55 (50) | 5-y HPV (78%) | 5-y HPV (28%) | <0.0001 | 5-y HPV (82%) | 5-y HPV (35%) | <0.0001 |

Abbreviations: HP, hypopharynx; L, larynx; n, number of patients tested for HPV status; N, total number of patients enrolled in the trial; Neg, negative; NP, nasopharynx; OC, oral cavity; OP, oropharynx; Pos, positive.

a Disease-specific survival.
b Failure-free survival.

MOVING FORWARD: HEAD AND NECK CLINICAL TRIAL DESIGN IN THE HPV ERA

Patients with HPV-positive tumors, therefore, are a clinically distinct subgroup within SCCHN. Study of such patients in future clinical trials requires consideration of several key issues:

1. How can current phase II trial data be reliably compared with historical controls?
2. How can HPV infection status best be incorporated into the statistical design of new phase III trials?
3. How is personalizing treatment for patients with favorable HPV-positive cancer and high-risk HPV-negative disease best addressed?

Issue 1: Control Data from Older Clinical Trials are Beset by New Confusion

This first issue stems from the increasing incidence of HPV infection and HPV-associated cancers in the context of decreased tobacco use.[2] The incidence of HPV-related cancer increased from 1973 to 2004 whereas the overall incidence of HPV-unrelated cancer declined. Many clinical trials were conducted between 1980 and 2000, and these trials continue to provide standard-of-care control treatments and reference data for calculation of statistical power and sample size for current trials. Tumor tissue samples from most of these trials are not available for HPV testing and it is difficult to accurately infer the HPV status based on the clinical characteristics, such as younger age, smoking history, and better performance status. It is difficult to directly apply results from these series to outcomes data generated from clinical trials performed in the HPV era.

Issue 2: New Clinical Trial Designs Must Directly Address HPV Infection Status

It is mandatory that patient enrollment in competing treatment arms of phase III trials be balanced for important prognostic characteristics to permit valid comparisons of treatment outcomes. Study arms containing unequal proportions of HPV-positive patients and HPV-negative patients with differing baseline relative risks for treatment failure would introduce severe bias and obscure final interpretation. For instance, if a phase III clinical trial is performed to study an experimental drug, this drug may falsely seem superior to current standard of care if the study cohort treated with the experimental drug contained more favorable-risk HPV-positive patients. In addition, difference in drug efficacy may be biased by either known or uncharacterized biologic differences between HPV-positive tumors and HPV-negative tumors. To categorically avoid these biases, growing consensus among investigators exists to support the opening of phase II/III trials that strictly study either HPV-positive disease or HPV-negative disease using HPV status as an integral biomarker.

Issue 3: Can Treatment Intensity Be Personalized According to HPV Infection Status to Improve Therapeutic Ratio?

Currently treatments of SCCHN have a severe impact on quality of life. Although aggressive radiotherapy and chemoradiotherapy regimens have improved survival outcomes,[15] such treatment yields severe post-treatment morbidity. Older radiotherapy techniques often resulted in restrictive fibrosis of the alimentary tract, which impaired swallowing and airway protection. Current intensity-modulated radiotherapy (IMRT) techniques permit protection of normal tissues adjacent to tumors[16,17] but still result in significant dysphagia and oral debilitation. Emerging data demonstrate that reducing the dose to the uninvolved larynx and pharyngeal axis improves post-treatment rehabilitation. Two reports based on prospectively gathered data demonstrate that modest reductions in radiation dose to oral cavity, superior pharyngeal constrictor muscles, and/or larynx are potentially associated with preserved long-term swallowing function.[18,19]

Thus, HPV-associated SCCOP represents a unique opportunity for carefully selected radiation dose shielding of novel dysphagia-specific anatomy to improve on-treatment therapeutic index and long-term quality of life. Additional focus has also been placed on reducing the overall intensity of combined modality treatment. It has been proposed that rational radiation dose reduction to responsive primary and nodal disease, coupled with avoidance of concurrent chemoradiotherapy, in patients triaged by induction chemotherapy to single-modality radiation in cases of complete response to induction is a promising approach. The rationale for use of induction chemotherapy is further strengthened by data confirming that the incidence of distant metastatic failure of HPV-positive disease is no lower than for high-risk HPV-negative disease.[9] Thus, this strategy has the potential to:

1. Reduce morbidity associated with concurrent chemoradiotherapy[20]
2. Improve systemic disease control through intensification of chemotherapy doses during the induction phase of treatment
3. Maintain gains in locoregional disease control in a patient population at low risk for such a failure pattern.[21]

Biomarkers: EGFR

HPV infection status has an impact on the potential utility of other candidate biomarkers of SCCHN outcomes. Tumor HPV status alone has limited relevance to non-oropharyngeal SCCHN, cannot discriminate prognosis with ideal specificity, and cannot predict outcomes for specific treatments. Fortunately, a growing list of complementary candidate biomarkers promises to improve predictive capability. A key example is epidermal growth factor receptor (EGFR), a cell-surface tyrosine kinase receptor critical to epithelial development and maintenance. Although some studies suggest poor prognosis after surgery or cytotoxic therapy in tumors with EGFR gene dosage,[22,23] this result has not been consistently reproduced[24,25] and has never been correlated with EGFR protein expression. A potentially more satisfying strategy would be to combine EGFR measures with mechanistically related markers of parallel signaling pathways[25–28] or HPV infection status in clinical head and neck tumor specimens.[29,30] Early studies suggested that HPV infection is inversely correlated with EGFR protein expression and that EGFR expression status may retain prognostic relevance regardless of HPV infection status. A more recent series has subsequently confirmed increased EGFR gene copy number status (as detected by fluorescence in situ hybridization) to remain largely confined to HPV-unassociated (eg, p16-negative) cancers.[31] Nonetheless, this study also showed that p16 expression supersedes EGFR-specific markers on multivariate analysis. Definitive prospective corroboration remains necessary but taken together these findings suggest a potential need to regularly combine at least HPV-specific and EGFR-specific biomarkers to guide future clinical strategies.

Imaging-based biomarkers: FDG-PET/CT

HPV infection status also has particular relevance to the ultimate utility of imaging-based biomarkers of SCCHN. Considerable interest has focused on fludeoxyglucose F 18 (FDG)–positron emission tomography (PET)/CT monitoring of SCCHN response to radiotherapy. Several groups have found that FDG-PET post-treatment restaging provides high negative predictive power[32–35]; accordingly, there is growing acceptance of withholding consolidative neck dissection after radiotherapy in the absence of residual FDG-avid adenopathy,[36] although some investigators argue that expert clinical interpretation of serial CT imaging could achieve similar results.[37,38] A potentially more effective and efficient approach would be to emphasize identification of specific clinical situations where FDG-PET/CT diagnostic yield may be optimized. FDG-PET/CT utility has been studied in the context of other important clinical parameters, in particular HPV infection status, through a bayesian, risk-based approach classically used by clinicians choosing between alternative diagnostic tests in specific patients. FDG-PET/CT seems to provide little value over CT alone in radiation response assessment for unselected patients with locally advanced SCCHN.[39,40] Nonetheless, FDG-PET/CT can significantly improve assessment of treatment response in high-risk patients, such as those with HPV-unassociated disease. These results provide critical impetus to incorporate risk-based stratification strategies informed of HPV infection status into FDG-PET/CT response assessment of locally advanced SCCHN. Such an individualized, context-specific approach will be relevant to any current or future imaging-based biomarker.

How Can These Issues Be Reconciled in Future Trials?

Currently ongoing trials that use HPV-positive status as an integral biomarker for eligibility criteria are summarized in **Table 3**. The first national cooperative group trial to test this concept is ECOG-E1308. This phase II study tests the role of induction chemotherapy followed by de-escalation of radiation dose and substitution of platinum chemotherapy with cetuximab. After the completion of induction chemotherapy, patients with complete response receive dose-reduced radiation with cetuximab. Patients with less than complete response receive standard curative doses of radiation with concurrent cetuximab. The RTOG has also opened a phase III clinical trial (RTOG 1016) directly comparing concurrent radiation/cisplatin with concurrent radiation/cetuximab. This trial will answer whether de-escalation of treatment away from conventional cytotoxic chemotherapy will result in decreased toxicity without compromising survival outcomes. There are several smaller institutional trials being conducted throughout North America and Europe designed to answer similar questions with varying approaches.

The concept of treatment de-escalation is not without controversy or risk. A recent retrospective study suggested that concurrent radiation and cetuximab is inferior to radiation and cisplatin.[41] Many investigators argue that the prognosis is favorable in patients with HPV-positive tumors because they are receiving full-dose radiation and chemotherapy. Although these patients have been observed to have favorable prognosis independent of the treatment modalities used, including chemotherapy, radiation, and/or surgery,[9–11,14,42] a subset of the HPV-positive patients experiences worse outcomes compared with average HPV-positive patients, resembling more of the clinical course of HPV-negative patients. This subset of patients has more-extensive smoking histories, TP53 mutations, and higher EGFR and Bcl-xL expressions, suggesting that the HPV status alone is not an adequate prognostic marker to perfectly segregate patients.[6,9,29] Current de-escalation trials do not stratify for these additional factors and could potentially undertreat a subset of patients. In addition, advances in minimally invasive surgical technique have brought primary surgical options to the table. The role of the currently available HPV vaccines for cancer prevention is another field of investigation. How best to treat these patients is the subject of ongoing discussion among clinical investigators and in clinical trial design. As in any clinical setting, when the treatment approach is not clear, these patients should be treated in the context of a clinical trial.

Table 3
Currently ongoing clinical trials using HPV or p16 status as an integral biomarker for the eligibility criteria of newly diagnosed, locally advanced, resectable oropharynx squamous cell carcinoma (ClinicalTrials.gov)

Study ID	NCI Trial ID	Trial Type	Total (N)	Treatment Arms	Primary Endpoint
E1308	NCT01084083	Phase II	160	Sequential therapy: cisplatin/paclitaxel/ cetuximab Complete response: IMRT (27 fractions) + cetuximab or noncomplete response: IMRT (33 fractions) + cetuximab	2-y PFS
J0988	NCT01088802	Phase I/II	60	IMRT (lower dose) + cisplatin	Toxicity, LRC
Dana-Farber Cancer Institute	NCT01221753	Phase II	50	Sequential therapy: docetaxel/cispplatin/ 5-fluorouracil Complete response: IMRT (lower dose) + carboplatin + cetuximab or noncomplete response: IMRT (full dose) + carboplatin + cetuximab	2-y and 5-y LRC
RTOG 1016	NCT01302834	Phase III	706	IMRT hyperfactionation + cisplatin vs IMRT hyperfactionation + cetuximab	5-y OS

Abbreviation: LRC, local-regional control.

Also at issue is the complementary problem of how best to personalize and improve outcomes for treatment of high-risk HPV-negative disease. Radiation response rates for patients with HPV-negative tumors are unacceptably low.[9–11,13] For instance, the authors' institutional data confirm a 44% complete response rate in HPV-negative oropharyngeal tumors versus 95% for HPV-positive tumors.[39] Radiation dose escalation is a potential strategy to improve control rates in this high-risk population, but bystander treatment of neighboring normal structures must be minimized to provide a feasible therapeutic ratio. The need for improved treatment outcomes for HPV-negative oropharyngeal cancer patients has motivated the authors' group to investigate the use of stereotactic radiosurgery (SRS) to escalate dose to HPV-unassociated primary disease, which serves as the most likely source for locoregional disease recurrence. SRS incorporates large single-dose treatment to overwhelm the capacity of radioresistant tumor cells to repair DNA damage and to incapacitate angiogenic stromal vessels, which supply these cells with oxygen and nutrients. SRS employs high-precision techniques to provide submillimeter precision to physically restrict high dose away from at-risk normal anatomy. In the head and neck region, such pertinent structures include central nervous system structures, mandible, muscles of mastication, salivary glands, larynx, oral cavity, mucosa, and pharyngeal constrictor muscles. Although promising in theory, use of SRS in this clinical context is novel and a formal phase I study is ongoing to carefully determine maximum tolerated treatment doses and optimal planning techniques for this approach.

SUMMARY

HPV-positive SCCOP and HPV-negative SCCOP represent discrete cancers, with differing biologic mechanisms, epidemiology, and natural history. The favorable responsiveness of HPV-positive SCCOP to current treatment represents an exciting opportunity for studying careful treatment deintensification to reduce acute toxicity and improve long-term patient recovery. These goals are well within grasp, because it potentially can be achieved with well-established clinical modalities, such as high-precision radiotherapy techniques, evolving surgical advances, and improved systemic treatment options. Through the collective effort of researchers and clinicians, personalized clinical trials incorporating HPV infection status promises to accelerate progress in treatment outcomes for SCCOP.

REFERENCES

1. Sturgis EM, Cinciripini PM. Trends in head and neck cancer incidence in relation to smoking prevalence: an emerging epidemic of human papillomavirus-associated cancers? Cancer 2007;110:1429–35.
2. Chaturvedi AK, Engels EA, Anderson WF, et al. Incidence trends for human papillomavirus-related and -unrelated oral squamous cell carcinomas in the United States. J Clin Oncol 2008;26:612–9.
3. Gillison ML, Koch WM, Capone RB, et al. Evidence for a causal association between human papillomavirus and a subset of head and neck cancers. J Natl Cancer Inst 2000;92:709–20.
4. D'Souza G, Kreimer AR, Viscidi R, et al. Case-control study of human papillomavirus and oropharyngeal cancer. N Engl J Med 2007;356:1944–56.
5. Fakhry C, Westra WH, Li S, et al. Improved survival of patients with human papillomavirus-positive head and neck squamous cell carcinoma in a prospective clinical trial. J Natl Cancer Inst 2008;100:261–9.
6. Worden FP, Kumar B, Lee JS, et al. Chemoselection as a strategy for organ preservation in advanced oropharynx cancer: response and survival positively associated with HPV16 copy number. J Clin Oncol 2008;26:3138–46.
7. Kies MS, Holsinger FC, Lee JJ, et al. Induction chemotherapy and cetuximab for locally advanced squamous cell carcinoma of the head and neck: results from a phase II prospective trial. J Clin Oncol 2010;28:8–14.
8. Cmelak AJ, Li S, Goldwasser MA, et al. Phase II trial of chemoradiation for organ preservation in resectable stage III or IV squamous cell carcinomas of the larynx or oropharynx: results of Eastern Cooperative Oncology Group Study E2399. J Clin Oncol 2007;25:3971–7.
9. Ang KK, Harris J, Wheeler R, et al. Human papillomavirus and survival of patients with oropharyngeal cancer. N Engl J Med 2010;363:24–35.
10. Lassen P, Eriksen JG, Hamilton-Dutoit S, et al. Effect of HPV-associated p16INK4A expression on response to radiotherapy and survival in squamous cell carcinoma of the head and neck. J Clin Oncol 2009;27:1992–8.
11. Lassen P, Eriksen JG, Hamilton-Dutoit S, et al. HPV-associated p16-expression and response to hypoxic modification of radiotherapy in head and neck cancer. Radiother Oncol 2009;94:30–5.

12. Lassen P, Eriksen JG, Krogdahl A, et al. The influence of HPV-associated p16-expression on accelerated fractionated radiotherapy in head and neck cancer: evaluation of the randomised DAHANCA 6&7 trial. Radiother Oncol 2011;100: 49–55.
13. Rischin D, Young RJ, Fisher R, et al. Prognostic significance of p16INK4A and human papillomavirus in patients with oropharyngeal cancer treated on TROG 02.02 phase III trial. J Clin Oncol 2010;28:4142–8.
14. Posner MR, Lorch JH, Goloubeva O, et al. Survival and human papillomavirus in oropharynx cancer in TAX 324: a subset analysis from an international phase III trial. Ann Oncol 2011;22:1071–7.
15. Argiris A. Update on chemoradiotherapy for head and neck cancer. Curr Opin Oncol 2002;14:323–9.
16. Chao KS. Protection of salivary function by intensity-modulated radiation therapy in patients with head and neck cancer. Semin Radiat Oncol 2002;12:20–5.
17. Chao KS, Wippold FJ, Ozyigit G, et al. Determination and delineation of nodal target volumes for head-and-neck cancer based on patterns of failure in patients receiving definitive and postoperative IMRT. Int J Radiat Oncol Biol Phys 2002;53: 1174–84.
18. Feng FY, Kim HM, Lyden TH, et al. Intensity-modulated chemoradiotherapy aiming to reduce dysphagia in patients with oropharyngeal cancer: clinical and functional results. J Clin Oncol 2010;28:2732–8.
19. Schwartz DL, Hutcheson K, Barringer D, et al. Candidate dosimetric predictors of long-term swallowing dysfunction after oropharyngeal intensity-modulated radiotherapy. Int J Radiat Oncol Biol Phys 2010;78:1356–65.
20. Trotti A, Bellm LA, Epstein JB, et al. Mucositis incidence, severity and associated outcomes in patients with head and neck cancer receiving radiotherapy with or without chemotherapy: a systematic literature review. Radiother Oncol 2003;66: 253–62.
21. Garden AS, Asper JA, Morrison WH, et al. Is concurrent chemoradiation the treatment of choice for all patients with Stage III or IV head and neck carcinoma? Cancer 2004;100:1171–8.
22. Chung CH, Ely K, McGavran L, et al. Increased epidermal growth factor receptor gene copy number is associated with poor prognosis in head and neck squamous cell carcinomas. J Clin Oncol 2006;24:4170–6.
23. Temam S, Kawaguchi H, El-Naggar AK, et al. Epidermal growth factor receptor copy number alterations correlate with poor clinical outcome in patients with head and neck squamous cancer. J Clin Oncol 2007;25:2164–70.
24. Freier K, Joos S, Flechtenmacher C, et al. Tissue microarray analysis reveals site-specific prevalence of oncogene amplifications in head and neck squamous cell carcinoma. Cancer Res 2003;63:1179–82.
25. Pectasides E, Rampias T, Kountourakis P, et al. Comparative prognostic value of epidermal growth factor quantitative protein expression compared with FISH for head and neck squamous cell carcinoma. Clin Cancer Res 2011;17:2947–54.
26. Grandis J, Melhem M, Gooding W, et al. Levels of TGF-alpha and EGFR protein in head and neck squamous cell carcinoma and patient survival. J Natl Cancer Inst 1998;90:824–32.
27. Barnes CJ, Ohshiro K, Rayala SK, et al. Insulin-like growth factor receptor as a therapeutic target in head and neck cancer. Clin Cancer Res 2007;13:4291–9.
28. Seiwert TY, Jagadeeswaran R, Faoro L, et al. The MET receptor tyrosine kinase is a potential novel therapeutic target for head and neck squamous cell carcinoma. Cancer Res 2009;69:3021–31.

29. Kumar B, Cordell KG, Lee JS, et al. EGFR, p16, HPV Titer, Bcl-xL and p53, sex, and smoking as indicators of response to therapy and survival in oropharyngeal cancer. J Clin Oncol 2008;26:3128–37.

30. Kong CS, Narasimhan B, Cao H, et al. The relationship between human papillomavirus status and other molecular prognostic markers in head and neck squamous cell carcinomas. Int J Radiat Oncol Biol Phys 2009;74:553–61.

31. Young RJ, Rischin D, Fisher R, et al. Relationship between epidermal growth factor receptor status, p16(INK4A), and outcome in head and neck squamous cell carcinoma. Cancer Epidemiol Biomarkers Prev 2011;20:1230–7.

32. Ryan WR, Fee WE Jr, Le QT, et al. Positron-emission tomography for surveillance of head and neck cancer. Laryngoscope 2005;115:645–50.

33. Yao M, Graham MM, Smith RB, et al. Value of FDG PET in assessment of treatment response and surveillance in head-and-neck cancer patients after intensity modulated radiation treatment: a preliminary report. Int J Radiat Oncol Biol Phys 2004;60:1410–8.

34. Porceddu SV, Jarmolowski E, Hicks RJ, et al. Utility of positron emission tomography for the detection of disease in residual neck nodes after (chemo)radiotherapy in head and neck cancer. Head Neck 2005;27:175–81.

35. Ong SC, Schoder H, Lee NY, et al. Clinical utility of 18F-FDG PET/CT in assessing the neck after concurrent chemoradiotherapy for Locoregional advanced head and neck cancer. J Nucl Med 2008;49:532–40.

36. Yao M, Hoffman HT, Chang K, et al. Is planned neck dissection necessary for head and neck cancer after intensity-modulated radiotherapy? Int J Radiat Oncol Biol Phys 2007;68:707–13.

37. Liauw SL, Mancuso AA, Amdur RJ, et al. Postradiotherapy neck dissection for lymph node-positive head and neck cancer: the use of computed tomography to manage the neck. J Clin Oncol 2006;24:1421–7.

38. Tan A, Adelstein DJ, Rybicki LA, et al. Ability of positron emission tomography to detect residual neck node disease in patients with head and neck squamous cell carcinoma after definitive chemoradiotherapy. Arch Otolaryngol Head Neck Surg 2007;133:435–40.

39. Moeller BJ, Rana V, Cannon BA, et al. Prospective imaging assessment of mortality risk after head-and-neck radiotherapy. Int J Radiat Oncol Biol Phys 2010;78:667–74.

40. Moeller BJ, Rana V, Cannon BA, et al. Prospective risk-adjusted [18F]Fluorodeoxyglucose positron emission tomography and computed tomography assessment of radiation response in head and neck cancer. J Clin Oncol 2009;27:2509–15.

41. Koutcher L, Sherman E, Fury M, et al. Concurrent cisplatin and radiation versus cetuximab and radiation for locally advanced head-and-neck cancer. Int J Radiat Oncol Biol Phys 2011;81(4):915–22.

42. Licitra L, Perrone F, Bossi P, et al. High-risk human papillomavirus affects prognosis in patients with surgically treated oropharyngeal squamous cell carcinoma. J Clin Oncol 2006;24:5630–6.

Biology of Human Papillomavirus Infection and Immune Therapy for HPV-Related Head and Neck Cancers

Simon R. Best, MD[a], Kevin J. Niparko, AB[b], Sara I. Pai, MD, PhD[a],*

KEYWORDS

- Vaccines • Immunotherapy • HPV-head and neck cancer • Oropharyngeal cancer

KEY POINTS

- Human papillomavirus (HPV)–related cancers result from the failure of the immune system to recognize and eliminate virus-infected cells.
- The lifetime exposure risk of HPV infection is high, but most individuals are able to clear the infection within 2 years.
- HPV-16 is one of the viral types to be cleared the slowest in men and is responsible for more than 90% of HPV-related head and neck cancers in the United States.
- Established HPV infections are naturally cleared through T-cell–mediated immune responses (CD4+ and CD8+ T cells) rather than humoral antibody responses.
- Therapeutic DNA vaccines induce T-cell responses against HPV-infected cells and, therefore, may play an important role in treating patients with established HPV-related diseases.

Key Abbreviations: BIOLOGY OF HPV INFECTION	
ACIP	Advisory Committee on Immunization Practices
CDC	Centers for Disease Control
CIN	Cervical intraepithelial neoplasia
CTL	Cytotoxic T lymphocyte
IFN	Interferon
IL	Interleukin
IRF	Interferon Regulatory Factor
mAb	Monoclonal antibody
MHC	Major histocompatibility complex
VLP	Viral like proteins
RRP	Recurrent respiratory papillomatosis

[a] Department of Otolaryngology-Head and Neck Surgery, Johns Hopkins School of Medicine, 601 North Caroline Street, JHOC 6th floor, Baltimore, MD 21287, USA; [b] Dartmouth College, Hanover, NH 03755, USA
* Corresponding author.
E-mail address: spai@jhmi.edu

Otolaryngol Clin N Am 45 (2012) 807–822
doi:10.1016/j.otc.2012.04.005
0030-6665/12/$ – see front matter © 2012 Elsevier Inc. All rights reserved.

INCIDENCE OF HUMAN PAPILLOMAVIRUS INFECTION

Human papillomavirus (HPV) infection is common in the general population, and the incidence varies by age and gender. The overall prevalence of HPV infection was 26.8% in a large cohort of women, and the prevalence increased to 44.8% among women aged 20 to 24 years.[1] In a prospective study designed to define the natural history of HPV infection in men, in a cohort of 1159 men, at least 1 type of HPV DNA was detected in 50% of men before enrollment and the incidence of new HPV infections during the study was 38.4/1000 person months over an average of 24 months.[2] The incidence of new infections in men was stable across all age groups, which differs significantly from women, in whom the incidence of new HPV infections decreases with increasing age.[3,4] This observation mirrors the declining prevalence of HPV infection in women past the peak prevalence in their mid-20s.[1]

Most HPV infections are cleared by the immune system within 2 years, defined as an absence of HPV DNA detection on follow-up serial swabs after detection of the initial infection.[2] At 12 months, 66% of infections are cleared; this increases to 90% at 24 months. However, in men, HPV-16 has been identified as one of the slowest viral types to be cleared, and takes nearly 2 times longer to be cleared than other high-risk viral types.[2] This is an interesting finding because HPV-16 is the viral type that accounts for more than 90% of HPV-related oropharyngeal cancers in the United States, and this disease is more prevalent in men than in women, suggesting possible gender differences in the ability to mount immunologic responses against this viral type.

Persistent oral HPV infection is a risk factor for the development of HPV-related oropharyngeal cancers. The prevalence of any HPV type in the oral cavity for both men and women is approximately 6.9%. However, when separated by gender, it is significantly higher in men (10%) than in women (3.6%).[5] Oral HPV infection is associated with certain sexual behaviors, with risk increasing with the number of lifetime oral sex partners.[6] In healthy individuals, the clearance rate for oral HPV infection at 6 months is approximately 40%.[7]

BIOLOGY OF HPV INFECTION

HPVs are small, nonenveloped DNA viruses with a double-stranded genome that encodes 6 early proteins (E1, E2, E3, E4, E5, E6, and E7) and 2 late proteins (L1 and L2), which are named based on their temporal expression pattern in the viral life cycle (**Fig. 1**).

Replication Cycle

The replication cycle of HPV has been well studied in the epithelium of the cervix, and has been found to be tightly linked to the differentiation of the epithelium that it infects. After infection of the undifferentiated epithelial cells within the basal cell layer, the E1 and E2 proteins are expressed and regulate viral replication and expression of the other early viral genes. As the infected cell migrates toward the superficial layers of the squamous epithelium, the E6 and E7 oncogenes are expressed and modify the cell cycle to retain the differentiating host keratinocyte in a state that is favorable for amplification of the viral genome. The E6 oncoprotein ubiquitinates p53, thereby flagging it for proteosomal degradation via the ubiquitin-proteasome pathway. The E7 protein competes for binding with E2F to the hypophosphorylated active form of the retinoblastoma tumor suppressor gene product, pRB, thus releasing the transcription factor E2F to bind and activate its targets to facilitate cell cycle progression. The binding affinity of E6 and E7 to p53 and pRB, respectively, differentiates the low and high risk types of HPV, which is based on the risk of the infected cell progressing to malignant transformation.

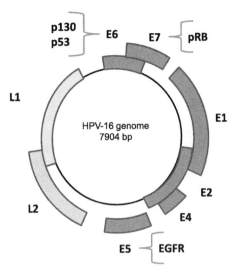

Fig. 1. HPV-16 genome. The circular HPV-16 genome is 7904 base pairs and encodes 6 early (E) and 2 late (L) major proteins. The primary cellular targets of these proteins are indicated on the genome diagram: E6 ubiquitinates p53, E7 competes for binding with E2F to the hypophosphorylated active form of retinoblastoma tumor suppressor gene product (pRB), and E5 upregulates EGFR.

Expression of Late Proteins

On cellular differentiation to the granular epithelial layer, the late proteins, L1 and L2, which consist of the major and minor capsid proteins respectively, are expressed and encapsulate the newly synthesized viral genomes. L1 spontaneously forms pentamers that assemble with the L2 protein to form the viral capsule.[8] These capsid proteins are linked by disulfide bonds to provide structural stability and protection against environmental insults when the virus is shed from the superficial epithelium.[9] The L2 protein is highly conserved among viral types, and is exposed during binding to a cell surface receptor during initial infection,[10] which completes the viral lifecycle.

Infection of Tonsils

In the head and neck region, HPV infects the basal cell layer of the reticulated squamous epithelium of the deep crypts within the lingual and palatine tonsils. The reticulated epithelium is a modified form of stratified squamous epithelium, which contains lymphocytes, plasma cells, macrophages, and interdigitating cells that migrate between the reticulated epithelium and underlying lymphoid stroma. Therefore, the basement membrane of the squamous epithelium lining the deep crypts is disrupted to allow for passage of lymphocytes and antigen-presenting cells from the external environment of the oropharynx to the tonsillar lymphoid tissue. Based on the function of the tonsil, its microanatomy leaves the basal cell layer vulnerable to HPV infection.

CELLULAR PROGRESSION TO DYSPLASIA AND CANCER

Many HPV infections are either cleared by the immune system or result in latent infections of the basal cell layer, with low viral copy numbers maintained indefinitely, or until injury or immunosuppression induces active infection. Integration of viral DNA into the host genome is a strong predictor of risk of progression from viral infection to neoplastic disease.[11] Late genes (L1 and L2) and some early genes (E1 and E2) are commonly deleted with viral integration and, with the disruption of E2 expression, there is unregulated expression of the E6 and E7 oncoproteins.[12,13] Concurrently, E5 upregulates the expression of epidermal growth factor receptor (EGFR) within the cell,[14] which leads to the overexpression of proto-oncogenes and repression of p21 (cyclin-dependent kinase inhibitor 1A) expression, a regulatory protein that controls cell apoptosis and differentiation.[14] The interruption of cellular mechanisms that regulate apoptosis and the cell cycle results in dysregulated cell cycle proliferation, delayed cellular differentiation, increased frequency of spontaneous and mutagen-induced mutations, and increased chromosomal instability.[15] Thus, the overexpression of the viral oncoproteins, E6 and E7, drives and maintains the neoplastic process.

IMMUNE SYSTEM AND HPV

Several lines of evidence highlight the importance of a functioning immune system in controlling HPV infection and its associated neoplasms:

1. Foremost is the observation that most immune-competent individuals infected with HPV are able to clear the infection without any clinical manifestation, and it is only 10% of infected individuals who develop HPV-related lesions.[2]
2. Histologic examination of spontaneously regressing HPV-related lesions shows infiltration of CD4+ and CD8+ T cells, whereas these immune cells are lacking in the lesions of patients with persistent disease.[16] Immunocompromised individuals such as organ transplant recipients on immunosuppressive medications[17] and patients infected with human immunodeficiency virus (HIV)[7] have been documented to have significantly increased rates of HPV infections and of HPV-related diseases.[18,19] Once these individuals stop their immunosuppressive medications or recover their immune cell counts, they are able to clear the infection and associated lesions.
3. Preclinical studies have reported that animals immunized with vaccines that elicit HPV-specific CD8+ T cells show regression of established HPV-related cancers.[20,21]

Humoral Immune Response

Clinically, systemic immune responses against HPV infection are often detected as humoral responses generated against the configured L1 pentamer, but this response is weak, inconsistent, and may not protect against future reinfection.[22] For high-risk types, the seroconversion rate is only 30% to 50% following documented infection[23] and, in patients with HPV-associated cancer, 30% to 50% have detectable antibody levels against the L1 protein from the causative viral type.[24] If present, the antibody titers can persist for many years even after the infection is cleared, so seropositivity is a useful marker for past infection rather than current infection.

Humoral immune responses to the early viral proteins have also been detected. Patients with cervical cancer can have detectable antibodies to E7[25] and patients who have HPV-related head and neck cancer have detectable antibodies to E6 (Dr Sara Pai, unpublished data, 2012). Serum analysis for antibodies against the full viral proteome therefore has promise as a screening method for HPV-associated oropharyngeal cancer.[26] However, patients with pure hypogammaglobulinemia seem to be at no higher risk of developing HPV-related diseases than patients with normal immune function, suggesting that humoral responses do not play a major role in clearing established HPV infections.

Cell-Mediated Immune Response

It is the cell-mediated immune responses, or HPV-specific CD4+ and CD8+ T cells, that are most critical in clearing established lesions (**Fig. 2**). The virus-specific CD4+ and CD8+ T cells coordinate to clear chronic viral infections,[27] and patients with evidence of previously cleared HPV-16 infections have strong detectable T-cell responses to viral proteins.[28] Deficits in T-cell response have been documented in patients with cervical cancer and in patients with cervical intraepithelial neoplasia.[29,30] The relative contributions to this lack of T-cell response from inherent host genetic factors[31] and/or viral mechanisms to escape immune recognition are not known.

VIRAL MECHANISMS TO EVADE THE IMMUNE SYSTEM

HPV has evolved multiple mechanisms to evade host immunologic responses,[32,33] thereby leading to successful establishment of HPV-related lesions.

Coordination of Viral Replication to Cellular Differentiation

The first adaptive mechanism for escaping immune surveillance is the coordination of viral replication to cellular differentiation.

In the uterine cervix, within the organization of stratified squamous epithelium, the degree of immune surveillance decreases considerably in the superficial, keratinized layers. HPV takes advantage of this organization by tightly regulating its own replication with differentiation of the keratinocyte. The virus evades cytotoxic T lymphocyte (CTL) responses by expressing a minimal level of viral gene products in the keratinocytes of the basal cell layer and upregulates expression of viral gene products with differentiation and upward migration of keratinocytes, away from areas of active immune

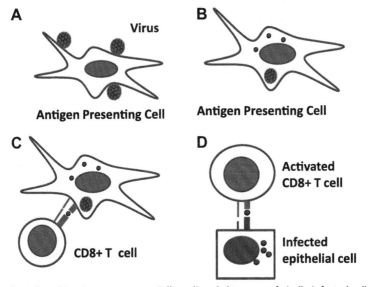

Fig. 2. Cell-mediated immune responses. Cell-mediated clearance of virally infected cells begins with (A) antigen-presenting cells encountering viral particles or proteins. (B) The virus is engulfed by the antigen-presenting cell and undergoes intracellular degradation. (C) The viral peptides are then presented to immature CD8+ T cells via major histocompatibility complex (MHC) class I molecules. (D) These activated cytotoxic CD8+ T cells then recognize and eliminate virally infected epithelial cells. (Data from Janeway C. Immunobiology. 5th edition. New York: Garland Publishing; 2001; and Male D, Brostoff J, Roth D; et al. Immunology. 7th edition. Philadelphia: Mosby, 2006.)

surveillance. In addition, HPV does not cause lysis of keratinocytes; virions are released through the mechanical breakage of surface epithelium and thereby minimize any associated inflammatory response. In this way, HPV replication is a local phenomenon with minimal systemic immune activation.

In the tonsil, HPV infects the reticulated epithelium lining the deep tonsillar crypts. Recent data suggest that the deep crypts of tonsils may be immune-privileged sites that can inhibit the effector function of HPV-specific T cells and thereby facilitate immune evasion at the time of initial HPV infection. This mechanism provides a biologic explanation of how a virus can infect a lymphoid organ, such as the tonsil and base of tongue, but still evade immune recognition and clearance (Lyford-Pike and colleagues, in preparation).

Inhibitory Effects of Viral Proteins

In addition to the local immunosuppressive microenvironment that HPV infects, the viral proteins also have local inhibitory effects on inflammatory cytokines to dampen both innate and adaptive immune responses. The HPV E5 and E7 proteins downregulate expression of the major histocompatibility complex (MHC) class I molecules, which inhibits viral antigen presentation to the immune system.[34,35] E6 and E7 have also been shown to reduce expression of Toll-like receptor 9[36] and cytokines, such as interleukin (IL)-8[37] and IL-18,[38] which are all potent proinflammatory molecules. A blunted response to interferon (IFN)-α and IFN-γ has also been observed in HPV infections.[39,40] One mechanism for the blunted response is a reduction in the expression of IFN regulatory factor 1 (IRF-1), which is a transcription factor that mediates IFN responses.[41] Because IFN signaling is a critical component in the activation of many aspects of both the innate and adaptive immune responses, as well as a potent antiproliferative agent, HPV thus disables a major mechanism of immune surveillance to oncogenic transformation.

PREVENTION OF HPV INFECTION THROUGH VACCINATION

Because the immune system is so important in controlling HPV infections and the lesions associated with these viruses, in the past decade vaccination programs against HPV have been initiated in the United States and other parts of the world.

Vaccines for the Prevention of Cancer

The discovery that the L1 viral proteins self-assemble into viral-like proteins (VLPs) in the absence of viral DNA was the critical first step in developing preventative vaccines.[42] Recombinant techniques could then be used to produce hollow VLPs that could induce protective L1 antibody levels that can protect against new HPV infection without the risk of being exposed to an infectious virus (**Fig. 3**).[43]

Quadrivalent VLP vaccine for girls and women
Large-scale trials to test the efficacy of this vaccination strategy were carried out in the early 2000s, and have led to the approval of 2 vaccines for the prevention of HPV-related diseases and cancers. A quadrivalent (HPV types 6/11/16/18) VLP vaccine was approved in June 2006 for administration to girls and women aged 9 to 26 years. Randomized, double-blinded, placebo-controlled trials evaluated the ability of the quadrivalent vaccine to prevent HPV-related anogenital diseases in women[44,45]: genital warts, vulvar, vaginal, cervical neoplasia (Females United to Unilaterally Reduce Endo/Ectocervical Disease [FUTURE I]); also high-grade cervical intraepithelial neoplasia (FUTURE II). The trials showed 100% protection against the development of anogenital lesions related to the 4 viral types. As a result, the Centers for Disease Control (CDC)

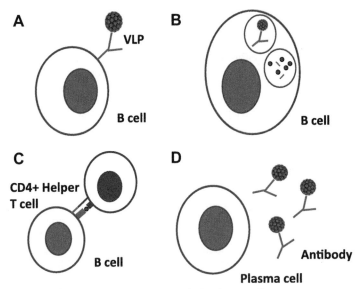

Fig. 3. Mechanism of preventative vaccines in inducing humoral immune responses after vaccination. The quadrivalent and bivalent HPV vaccines consist of the L1 capsid protein, which self-assembles into VLPs. The humoral immune system is activated by (*A*) recognition of the VLPs by a B-cell surface immunoglobulin. (*B*) The VLP is internalized and degraded into peptides, which (*C*) are then presented to CD4+ helper T cells via MHC class II molecules. (*D*) An activated B cell then proliferates and differentiates into an antibody-secreting plasma cell. These circulating antibodies then recognize and bind HPV to prevent viral infection of an epithelial cell. (*Data from* Janeway C. Immunobiology. 5th edition. New York: Garland Publishing; 2001; and Male D, Brostoff J, Roth D; et al. Immunology. 7th edition. Philadelphia: Mosby, 2006.)

Advisory Committee on Immunization Practices (ACIP) in 2007 recommended vaccination for all girls ages 11 to 12 years, before the age of sexual debut and the risk of exposure to HPV.

Bivalent VLP vaccine for girls and women
A second prophylactic bivalent (HPV types 16/18) VLP vaccine was approved in October of 2009 for use in girls and women aged 10 to 25 years. Although this vaccine does not include HPV types 6 and 11, a head-to-head clinical trial showed that the bivalent vaccine induced higher antibody titers against the high-risk viral types compared to the quadrivalent vaccine.[46] Both of these vaccines are given as 3 doses administered over a 6-month period. The length of protection against HPV infection achieved through these vaccines is currently being studied to determine whether booster vaccinations will be required to maintain immune protection against HPV.

Quadrivalent vaccine for boys and men
In October of 2009, the quadrivalent vaccine was approved for boys and men aged 9 to 26 years. A randomized, placebo-controlled, double-blinded trial reported on the safety of the quadrivalent vaccine and on its efficacy in preventing the development of HPV-related external anogenital lesions in boys and men.[47] The study enrolled 4065 healthy boys and men between 16 and 26 years of age across 18 countries. There was a per-protocol population in which subjects were documented to be negative for exposure to the HPV types at the time of enrollment and these subjects received all 3 vaccinations. The intention-to-treat

population included subjects whose baseline HPV exposure history was unknown and these subjects received either the vaccine or placebo. The study reported that the quadrivalent vaccine efficacy was 90.4% against the development of genital lesions related to the HPV-6, HPV-11, HPV-16, or HPV-18 viral types in HPV-naïve patients and the efficacy decreased to 65.5% in patients with an unknown HPV exposure history. Based on these study results, in October 2011, the CDC ACIP recommended that boys aged 11 to 12 years receive the vaccine. These studies show that there is benefit to vaccinating both boys and girls. However, the benefits of the HPV vaccine will not be appreciated for several decades, and it is unclear how the vaccine will affect oral mucosal immunity or oral HPV infection and, thus, the development of HPV-related head and neck cancers.

Implementation of Vaccination and the Elimination of Population Risk

To eradicate HPV, a herd immunization strategy would need to be implemented. However, even with strong governmental recommendations for HPV vaccination, there are many sociologic and logistical factors that make this goal challenging. A nationwide survey of girls aged 13 to 17 years by the CDC in 2010 found that less than half (48.7%) had received at least 1 dose of the 3-part HPV vaccination series and, of the teenagers who commenced the vaccination series, 30% did not complete the series.[48] There are several reasons that are thought to account for the low vaccination rates, including some parents' misconception that giving the vaccine promotes sexual activity, associated high vaccine costs ($130 for the series), as well as delivery costs, lack of insurance coverage for vaccination, the requirement for obtaining 3 doses of vaccine over a 6-month period, inability to reach out to this target population because it has not previously been served by immunization programs.

As increasing numbers of boys and girls receive the vaccine, the overall prevalence of HPV and its associated diseases in the population should decrease, indirectly benefiting those who may not have been vaccinated. Using disease modeling of the 14 high-risk HPV types, it is estimated that, if 50% of women are vaccinated against HPV-16/18, there would be a 47% reduction in cervical cancer, with 25% of the prevented cases occurring in women who never received the vaccine.[49] With more than 20 million Americans currently infected with HPV in the United States, and an estimated 6 million new infections to occur each year,[50] vaccination programs, when implemented, have great potential to reduce the burden of HPV disease and to prevent its related cancers.

As stated previously, the impact of current prophylactic vaccines on HPV-associated oropharyngeal cancer is unknown. As vaccination programs decrease the overall prevalence of HPV infection in the population, the trends of increasing oropharyngeal cancer[51] may show signs of slowing or even reversing. However, none of the prophylactic vaccine studies performed thus far have evaluated oral HPV infection or oral immunity to HPV, so its impact on the incidence of HPV-associated oropharyngeal cancer remains an open question.

IMMUNOTHERAPY FOR THE TREATMENT OF ESTABLISHED HPV-ASSOCIATED DISEASE

The vaccination strategies discussed have focused on preventing viral infection of epithelial cells through the generation of antibody responses that recognize the viral capsid proteins. However, this strategy is not effective for treating existing infections or established HPV-related diseases. Treatment of established disease requires activation of the cellular immune system, both CD4+ and CD8+ T cells, which can recognize and eliminate virus-infected cells. The differences between preventative and therapeutic vaccine strategies are outlined in **Table 1**.

Table 1
Differences between prophylactic and therapeutic vaccines

	Prophylactic Vaccine	Therapeutic Vaccine
Prevent new infection	Yes	No
Treat existing infection	No	Yes
Effector cells	B cells	CD4+ T cells, CD8+ T cells
Humoral (antibody) response	High	Low
Cell-mediated (T cell) response	Low	High
Vaccine construction	Whole organism: live/attenuated/killed; protein subunits	DNA plasmid; peptides/proteins Dendritic cell
Targeted antigen	Cell surface viral capsid protein	Intracellular viral protein

Immunotherapy for the Treatment of Cancer

In developing therapeutic vaccination strategies, the identification of tumor-specific antigens determines the specificity of the targeted immune response. The HPV E6 and E7 proteins represent such model tumor antigens for several reasons. These oncoproteins are foreign viral proteins and, thus, are more immunogenic than a self-protein, which may be mutated in the cancer cell, such as p53, or aberrantly upregulated, such as Mage-A3. The proteins are encoded by the viral genome and are uniquely expressed by all virus-infected cell and, thus, every virus-related cancer cell. Because the E6 and E7 oncoproteins are required for the induction and maintenance of the malignant phenotype, these proteins are constitutively expressed within the cancer cells and it is unlikely that the cancer cell would downregulate expression of these proteins to evade an immunologic response.

Therapeutic Vaccines for HPV

One group developed a therapeutic HPV vaccine that consisted of synthetic long peptides that spanned both the HPV-16 E6 and E7 proteins. A phase II clinical trial was completed in 20 women with HPV-16–associated grade III vulvar intraepithelial neoplasia (VIN).[52] The patients were vaccinated with these overlapping peptides every 3 weeks for a total for 4 vaccinations. Biopsies were performed at 3 and 12 months after the last vaccination. All patients mounted vaccine-induced immune responses and clinical responses correlated with the induction of HPV-16–specific CD8+ T cells. Most immune responses were specific to the HPV-16 E6 protein. A complete response was observed in 25% (5/20) of patients 3 months after the last vaccination, and this increased to a 47% (9/19) complete response rate 12 months after the last vaccination. This study showed for the first time that, with vaccination, complete response rates could be achieved for established HPV disease.

In addition to peptide-based and protein-based vaccines, several groups have evaluated DNA vaccines that allow for continued, high levels of target gene expression in transfected cells and, thus, sustained immunologic responses. HPV DNA vaccines have been evaluated in clinical trials for HPV-associated diseases such as cervical intraepithelial neoplasia (CIN)[53] and also are being evaluated in HPV-related head and neck cancers in an ongoing clinical trial.[54]

Strategies to Enhance Therapeutic Vaccines

One of the challenges with immunotherapy and therapeutic vaccination is generating a robust and relevant T-cell response specific to the antigen of interest. Therefore, various strategies for increasing the immunogenicity of vaccines have been evaluated in the development of DNA vaccines. For example:

- The target antigen can be linked to chaperone proteins that target the tumor antigen to cellular pathways, which enhances its presentation to the immune system.[55]
- The DNA vaccine can also be administered using electroporation, or via a gene gun, rather than traditional intramuscular needle injection, which can significantly enhance the levels of antigen expression within the cell and/or increase the transfection rate of dendritic cells within the skin milieu.[20]
- Combining vaccination with chemotherapeutic agents can also enhance the immune response by inducing tumor cell apoptosis and inflammation, which broadens tumor antigen presentation to the immune system.[56]

All of these strategies to enhance the efficacy of HPV DNA vaccines, in addition to others, are currently being investigated in the treatment of HPV-associated head and neck cancers.[54]

OTHER MOLECULAR TARGETS FOR THE TREATMENT OF HPV-ASSOCIATED DISEASE

Although the E6 and E7 oncoproteins are the most common immunotherapeutic targets in HPV-associated cancers, the virus alters other cellular pathways that can be targeted by nonimmunologic methods.

EGFR is highly expressed in a large percentage of head and neck cancers[57] and a monoclonal antibody against the receptor (cetuximab) has been found to have clinical efficacy in head and neck cancer.[58] The HPV-16 viral protein E5, in particular, has effects on EGFR trafficking in the cell and enhances EGFR pathway activation.[59,60] Increased EGFR expression is also seen in recurrent respiratory papillomatosis, a disease caused by HPV types 6 and 11.[61,62] There is an ongoing clinical trial for HPV-associated oropharyngeal cancer using induction chemotherapy followed by cetuximab with either reduced or standard-dose radiation.[63] The goal of the study is to determine whether comparable outcomes for HPV-associated cancer can be achieved with less intensive radiation by targeting EGFR. However, the interaction between these risk factors is not completely understood, since HPV positivity portends a good outcome in oropharyngeal cancer,[64] whereas EGFR expression is an independent risk factor for poor prognosis in head and neck cancer.[65]

Vascular endothelial growth factor (VEGF) has been implicated in many tumors as a promoter of tumor angiogenesis. There is evidence that HPV-16 E6 and E7 can upregulate VEGF expression,[66,67] and that E5 increases VEGF expression through the EGFR pathway.[68] This finding has relevance because a commercially available inhibitor of VEGF (bevacizumab) is on the market, although there have been no clinical studies to date to evaluate its use in HPV-associated oropharyngeal cancer.

In addition, there are 2 ongoing clinical trials evaluating Celebrex (celecoxib) to treat HPV-associated disease (cervical intraepithelial neoplasia[69] and recurrent respiratory papillomatosis [RRP]).[70] These studies are based on the observation that the COX-2 enzyme is overexpressed in HPV-related precancerous cervical lesions[71] as well as in RRP.[72] These studies highlight that targeted therapy against HPV-associated oropharyngeal cancers need not be limited to the viral oncoproteins themselves but also to downstream cellular pathways that may be altered based on viral protein expression within the cell.

CHALLENGES AND FUTURE DIRECTIONS OF IMMUNOTHERAPY FOR HPV-ASSOCIATED CANCERS

Although targeted immunotherapeutic strategies have great promise in the treatment of HPV-associated disease, significant challenges remain. The role of regulatory T cells in contributing to a local immunosuppressive microenvironment and in suppressing cytotoxic T-cell function in cancers is increasingly being appreciated.[73] The function of these regulatory T cells is to modulate activated T-cell function to prevent autoimmunity. However, in the setting of cancer immunotherapy, the regulatory T cells can dampen the desired vaccine-induced T-cell responses. Both HPV-related tumors and other cancers have populations of regulatory (FOXP3+) T cells and the presence of this T-cell population can predict lack of clinical response to therapeutic vaccination against HPV-16.[74] Therefore, groups have evaluated the combination of chemotherapeutic agents, such as cyclophosphamide, and cancer vaccines to eliminate the regulatory T-cell population to enhance vaccine-specific immune responses.[75]

In addition, antigen-induced activation and proliferation of T cells are regulated by the temporal expression and binding of both costimulatory and coinhibitory receptors. The orchestrated signaling through these receptors in adaptive cellular immunity modulates the initiation, escalation, and subsequent resolution of host immune responses. In the absence of coinhibitory signaling, persistent T-cell activation can lead to excessive tissue damage in the setting of infection as well as autoimmunity. In the context of cancer immunology, in which immune responses are directed against antigens specifically or selectively expressed by cancer cells, these immune checkpoints can represent major obstacles to overcoming tumor-specific tolerance and generating clinically meaningful tumor control. Therefore, efforts have been made in the clinical arena to investigate blockade of immune checkpoints as novel therapeutic approaches to cancer.

Two such coinhibitory T-cell receptors that are the focus of intense current interest are:

1. CTLA-4
2. Programmed cell death-1 (PD-1).

Ipilimumab, a monoclonal antibody (mAb) that blocks CTLA-4, was evaluated in patients with advanced metastatic melanoma in a randomized phase III clinical trial and showed a survival benefit; however, it was associated with significant immune-related toxicities.[76]

In a phase I clinical trial, a blocking mAb against PD-1 (MDX-1106) was evaluated in patients with advanced metastatic melanoma, colorectal cancer, castration-resistant prostate cancer, non–small cell lung cancer, and renal cell carcinoma. Blocking the PD-1 immune checkpoint seemed to be better tolerated than CTLA-4 blockade and, although the study was primarily a safety study, clinical activity was observed in all of the evaluated histologies except for prostate cancer.[77] Furthermore, tumor cell surface, or membranous expression of the major PD-1 ligand PD-L1 (also termed B7-H1) seemed to correlate with the likelihood of response to therapy. Future studies need to focus on characterizing the gene signatures of tumor immune infiltrates, to identify the factors responsible for inducing local immunosuppression within the tumor microenvironment.

SUMMARY

HPV is a ubiquitous virus that causes a wide range of human diseases, including a growing subset of oropharyngeal carcinomas. Significant progress has been made within the past decade in designing and implementing preventative vaccination programs against HPV. However, there are a variety of societal and economic challenges in implementing these vaccination programs, and the burden of HPV and its related cancers will continue until these challenges are addressed. Therefore, therapeutic vaccines need to be developed to treat those individuals already infected and/or diagnosed with established HPV-related disease. However, a different set of challenges are uncovered with therapeutic vaccines based on the biology of these tumors. As knowledge of cancer immunology matures, the obstacles to achieving successful immunotherapy are being revealed and strategies are being applied to address these barriers. The unharnessed potential of immunotherapy in treating virus-related cancers will undoubtedly be realized in the near future.

REFERENCES

1. Dunne EF, Unger ER, Sternberg M, et al. Prevalence of HPV infection among females in the United States. JAMA 2007;297(8):813–9.
2. Giuliano AR, Lee JH, Fulp W, et al. Incidence and clearance of genital human papillomavirus infection in men (HIM): a cohort study. Lancet 2011;377(9769): 932–40.
3. Castle PE, Schiffman M, Herrero R, et al. A prospective study of age trends in cervical human papillomavirus acquisition and persistence in Guanacaste, Costa Rica. J Infect Dis 2005;191(11):1808–16.
4. Munoz N, Mendez F, Posso H, et al. Incidence, duration, and determinants of cervical human papillomavirus infection in a cohort of Colombian women with normal cytological results. J Infect Dis 2004;190(12):2077–87.
5. Gillison ML, Broutian T, Pickard RK, et al. Prevalence of oral HPV Infection in the United States, 2009-2010. JAMA 2012;307(7):693–703.
6. D'Souza G, Agrawal Y, Halpern J, et al. Oral sexual behaviors associated with prevalent oral human papillomavirus infection. J Infect Dis 2009;199(9): 1263–9.
7. D'Souza G, Fakhry C, Sugar EA, et al. Six-month natural history of oral versus cervical human papillomavirus infection. Int J Cancer 2007;121(1):143–50.
8. Buck CB, Cheng N, Thompson CD, et al. Arrangement of L2 within the papillomavirus capsid. J Virol 2008;82(11):5190–7.
9. Buck CB, Thompson CD, Pang YY, et al. Maturation of papillomavirus capsids. J Virol 2005;79(5):2839–46.
10. Kines RC, Thompson CD, Lowy DR, et al. The initial steps leading to papillomavirus infection occur on the basement membrane prior to cell surface binding. Proc Natl Acad Sci U S A 2009;106(48):20458–63.
11. Peitsaro P, Johansson B, Syrjanen S. Integrated human papillomavirus type 16 is frequently found in cervical cancer precursors as demonstrated by a novel quantitative real-time PCR technique. J Clin Microbiol 2002;40(3):886–91.
12. Lazo PA. The molecular genetics of cervical carcinoma. Br J Cancer 1999;80(12): 2008–18.
13. Pett M, Coleman N. Integration of high-risk human papillomavirus: a key event in cervical carcinogenesis? J Pathol 2007;212(4):356–67.
14. Ragin CC, Modugno F, Gollin SM. The epidemiology and risk factors of head and neck cancer: a focus on human papillomavirus. J Dent Res 2007;86(2):104–14.
15. Howley PM. Role of the human papillomaviruses in human cancer. Cancer Res 1991;51(Suppl 18):5019s–22s.
16. Bourgault Villada I, Moyal Barracco M, Ziol M, et al. Spontaneous regression of grade 3 vulvar intraepithelial neoplasia associated with human

papillomavirus-16-specific CD4(+) and CD8(+) T-cell responses. Cancer Res 2004;64(23):8761–6.

17. Paternoster DM, Cester M, Resente C, et al. Human papilloma virus infection and cervical intraepithelial neoplasia in transplanted patients. Transplant Proc 2008; 40(6):1877–80.
18. Fruchter RG, Maiman M, Sedlis A, et al. Multiple recurrences of cervical intraepithelial neoplasia in women with the human immunodeficiency virus. Obstet Gynecol 1996;87(3):338–44.
19. Moscicki AB, Ellenberg JH, Farhat S, et al. Persistence of human papillomavirus infection in HIV-infected and -uninfected adolescent girls: risk factors and differences, by phylogenetic type. J Infect Dis 2004;190(1):37–45.
20. Best SR, Peng S, Juang CM, et al. Administration of HPV DNA vaccine via electroporation elicits the strongest CD8 + T cell immune responses compared to intramuscular injection and intradermal gene gun delivery. Vaccine 2009; 27(40):5450–9.
21. Cheng WF, Hung CF, Chai CY, et al. Tumor-specific immunity and antiangiogenesis generated by a DNA vaccine encoding calreticulin linked to a tumor antigen. J Clin Invest 2001;108(5):669–78.
22. Frazer IH. Interaction of human papillomaviruses with the host immune system: a well evolved relationship. Virology 2009;384(2):410–4.
23. Carter JJ, Koutsky LA, Hughes JP, et al. Comparison of human papillomavirus types 16, 18, and 6 capsid antibody responses following incident infection. J Infect Dis 2000;181(6):1911–9.
24. Carter JJ, Madeleine MM, Shera K, et al. Human papillomavirus 16 and 18 L1 serology compared across anogenital cancer sites. Cancer Res 2001;61(5): 1934–40.
25. Jochmus-Kudielka I, Schneider A, Braun R, et al. Antibodies against the human papillomavirus type 16 early proteins in human sera: correlation of anti-E7 reactivity with cervical cancer. J Natl Cancer Inst 1989;81(22):1698–704.
26. Anderson KS, Wong J, D'Souza G, et al. Serum antibodies to the HPV16 proteome as biomarkers for head and neck cancer. Br J Cancer 2011;104(12): 1896–905.
27. Matloubian M, Concepcion RJ, Ahmed R. CD4+ T cells are required to sustain CD8+ cytotoxic T-cell responses during chronic viral infection. J Virol 1994; 68(12):8056–63.
28. Welters MJ, de Jong A, van den Eeden SJ, et al. Frequent display of human papillomavirus type 16 E6-specific memory T-helper cells in the healthy population as witness of previous viral encounter. Cancer Res 2003;63(3): 636–41.
29. de Jong A, van Poelgeest MI, van der Hulst JM, et al. Human papillomavirus type 16-positive cervical cancer is associated with impaired CD4+ T-cell immunity against early antigens E2 and E6. Cancer Res 2004;64(15):5449–55.
30. Nakagawa M, Stites DP, Farhat S, et al. Cytotoxic T lymphocyte responses to E6 and E7 proteins of human papillomavirus type 16: relationship to cervical intraepithelial neoplasia. J Infect Dis 1997;175(4):927–31.
31. Hemminki K, Chen B. Familial risks for cervical tumors in full and half siblings: etiologic apportioning. Cancer Epidemiol Biomarkers Prev 2006;15(7):1413–4.
32. Tindle RW. Immune evasion in human papillomavirus-associated cervical cancer. Nat Rev Cancer 2002;2(1):59–65.
33. Stanley M. Immune responses to human papillomavirus. Vaccine 2006;24(Suppl 1): S16–22.

34. Woodworth CD. HPV innate immunity. Front Biosci 2002;7:d2058–71.
35. Ashrafi GH, Haghshenas MR, Marchetti B, et al. E5 protein of human papilloma-virus type 16 selectively downregulates surface HLA class I. Int J Cancer 2005; 113(2):276–83.
36. Hasan UA, Bates E, Takeshita F, et al. TLR9 expression and function is abolished by the cervical cancer-associated human papillomavirus type 16. J Immunol 2007; 178(5):3186–97.
37. Huang SM, McCance DJ. Down regulation of the interleukin-8 promoter by human papillomavirus type 16 E6 and E7 through effects on CREB binding protein/p300 and P/CAF. J Virol 2002;76(17):8710–21.
38. Lee SJ, Cho YS, Cho MC, et al. Both E6 and E7 oncoproteins of human papillo-mavirus 16 inhibit IL-18-induced IFN-gamma production in human peripheral blood mononuclear and NK cells. J Immunol 2001;167(1):497–504.
39. Barnard P, McMillan NA. The human papillomavirus E7 oncoprotein abrogates signaling mediated by interferon-alpha. Virology 1999;259(2):305–13.
40. Li S, Labrecque S, Gauzzi MC, et al. The human papilloma virus (HPV)-18 E6 on-coprotein physically associates with Tyk2 and impairs Jak-STAT activation by interferon-alpha. Oncogene 1999;18(42):5727–37.
41. Nees M, Geoghegan JM, Hyman T, et al. Papillomavirus type 16 oncogenes downregulate expression of interferon-responsive genes and upregulate proliferation-associated and NF-kappaB-responsive genes in cervical keratino-cytes. J Virol 2001;75(9):4283–96.
42. Zhou J, Sun XY, Stenzel DJ, et al. Expression of vaccinia recombinant HPV 16 L1 and L2 ORF proteins in epithelial cells is sufficient for assembly of HPV virion-like particles. Virology 1991;185(1):251–7.
43. Lowy DR, Schiller JT. Prophylactic human papillomavirus vaccines. J Clin Invest 2006;116(5):1167–73.
44. Garland SM, Hernandez-Avila M, Wheeler CM, et al. Quadrivalent vaccine against human papillomavirus to prevent anogenital diseases. N Engl J Med 2007;356(19):1928–43.
45. FUTURE II Study Group. Quadrivalent vaccine against human papilloma-virus to prevent high-grade cervical lesions. N Engl J Med 2007;356(19): 1915–27.
46. GlaxoSmithKline. Clinical trial NCT00423046. cited 2012. Available at: http:// clinicaltrials.gov/ct2/show/NCT00423046. Accessed May 24, 2012.
47. Giuliano AR, Palefsky JM, Goldstone S, et al. Efficacy of quadrivalent HPV vaccine against HPV Infection and disease in males. N Engl J Med 2011; 364(5):401–11.
48. CDC. National and state vaccination coverage among adolescents aged 13 through 17 years — United States, 2010. MMWR Morb Mortal Wkly Rep 2011; 117(60):1117–23.
49. Bogaards JA, Coupe VM, Xiridou M, et al. Long-term impact of human papilloma-virus vaccination on infection rates, cervical abnormalities, and cancer incidence. Epidemiology 2011;22(4):505–15.
50. CDC. Genital HPV infection - fact sheet 2011. Available at: http://www.cdc.gov/ std/hpv/stdfact-hpv.htm. Accessed May 24, 2012.
51. Chaturvedi AK, Engels EA, Pfeiffer RM, et al. Human papillomavirus and rising oropharyngeal cancer incidence in the United States. J Clin Oncol 2011; 29(32):4294–301.
52. Kenter GG, Welters MJ, Valentijn AR, et al. Vaccination against HPV-16 oncopro-teins for vulvar intraepithelial neoplasia. N Engl J Med 2009;361(19):1838–47.

53. Trimble CL, Peng S, Kos F, et al. A phase I trial of a human papillomavirus DNA vaccine for HPV16+ cervical intraepithelial neoplasia 2/3. Clin Cancer Res 2009;15(1):361–7.
54. Sidney Kimmel Comprehensive Cancer Center. Clinical trial NCT01493154 - Safety Study of HPV DNA Vaccine to Treat Head and Neck Cancer Patients. Available at: http://clinicaltrials.gov/ct2/show/NCT01493154. Accessed May 24, 2012.
55. Cheng WF, Hung CF, Chen CA, et al. Characterization of DNA vaccines encoding the domains of calreticulin for their ability to elicit tumor-specific immunity and antiangiogenesis. Vaccine 2005;23(29):3864–74.
56. Tseng CW, Hung CF, Alvarez RD, et al. Pretreatment with cisplatin enhances E7-specific CD8+ T-cell-mediated antitumor immunity induced by DNA vaccination. Clin Cancer Res 2008;14(10):3185–92.
57. Modjtahedi H. Molecular therapy of head and neck cancer. Cancer Metastasis Rev 2005;24(1):129–46.
58. Bonner JA, Harari PM, Giralt J, et al. Radiotherapy plus cetuximab for squamous-cell carcinoma of the head and neck. N Engl J Med 2006;354(6):567–78.
59. Pim D, Collins M, Banks L. Human papillomavirus type 16 E5 gene stimulates the transforming activity of the epidermal growth factor receptor. Oncogene 1992; 7(1):27–32.
60. Crusius K, Auvinen E, Steuer B, et al. The human papillomavirus type 16 E5-protein modulates ligand-dependent activation of the EGF receptor family in the human epithelial cell line HaCaT. Exp Cell Res 1998;241(1):76–83.
61. Lyford-Pike S, Westra WH, Loyo M, et al. Differential expression of epidermal growth factor receptor in juvenile and adult-onset recurrent respiratory papillomatosis. Histopathology 2010;57(5):768–70.
62. Johnston D, Hall H, DiLorenzo TP, et al. Elevation of the epidermal growth factor receptor and dependent signaling in human papillomavirus-infected laryngeal papillomas. Cancer Res 1999;59(4):968–74.
63. NCI. Clinical Trial NCT01084083 - Paclitaxel, cisplatin, and cetuximab followed by cetuximab and intensity-modulated radiation therapy in treating patients with HPV-associated stage III or stage IV cancer of the oropharynx that can be removed by surgery. Available at: http://clinicaltrials.gov/ct2/show/NCT01084083. Accessed May 24, 2012.
64. Ang KK, Harris J, Wheeler R, et al. Human papillomavirus and survival of patients with oropharyngeal cancer. N Engl J Med 2010;363(1):24–35.
65. Hong A, Dobbins T, Lee CS, et al. Relationships between epidermal growth factor receptor expression and human papillomavirus status as markers of prognosis in oropharyngeal cancer. Eur J Cancer 2010;46(11):2088–96.
66. Lopez-Ocejo O, Viloria-Petit A, Bequet-Romero M, et al. Oncogenes and tumor angiogenesis: the HPV-16 E6 oncoprotein activates the vascular endothelial growth factor (VEGF) gene promoter in a p53 independent manner. Oncogene 2000;19(40):4611–20.
67. Walker J, Smiley LC, Ingram D, et al. Expression of human papillomavirus type 16 E7 is sufficient to significantly increase expression of angiogenic factors but is not sufficient to induce endothelial cell migration. Virology 2011;410(2): 283–90.
68. Kim SH, Juhnn YS, Kang S, et al. Human papillomavirus 16 E5 up-regulates the expression of vascular endothelial growth factor through the activation of epidermal growth factor receptor, MEK/ ERK1,2 and PI3K/Akt. Cell Mol Life Sci 2006;63(7–8):930–8.

69. NCI. Clinical trial NCT00081263 - Celecoxib in treating patients with cervical intra-epithelial neoplasia. Available at: http://clinicaltrials.gov/ct2/show/NCT00081263. Accessed May 24, 2012.

70. North Shore Long Island Jewish Health System. Clinical trial NCT00571701 - Study of Celebrex (celecoxib) in patients with recurrent respiratory papillomatosis. Available at: http://clinicaltrials.gov/ct2/show/NCT00571701. Accessed May 24, 2012.

71. Saldivar JS, Lopez D, Feldman RA, et al. COX-2 overexpression as a biomarker of early cervical carcinogenesis: a pilot study. Gynecol Oncol 2007;107(1 Suppl 1): S155–62.

72. Wu R, Coniglio SJ, Chan A, et al. Up-regulation of Rac1 by epidermal growth factor mediates COX-2 expression in recurrent respiratory papillomas. Mol Med 2007;13(3–4):143–50.

73. Loddenkemper C, Hoffmann C, Stanke J, et al. Regulatory (FOXP3+) T cells as target for immune therapy of cervical intraepithelial neoplasia and cervical cancer. Cancer Sci 2009;100(6):1112–7.

74. Welters MJ, Kenter GG, de Vos van Steenwijk PJ, et al. Success or failure of vaccination for HPV16-positive vulvar lesions correlates with kinetics and phenotype of induced T-cell responses. Proc Natl Acad Sci U S A 2010;107(26): 11895–9.

75. Emens LA, Asquith JM, Leatherman JM, et al. Timed sequential treatment with cyclophosphamide, doxorubicin, and an allogeneic granulocyte-macrophage colony-stimulating factor-secreting breast tumor vaccine: a chemotherapy dose-ranging factorial study of safety and immune activation. J Clin Oncol 2009;27(35):5911–8.

76. Hodi FS, O'Day SJ, McDermott DF, et al. Improved survival with ipilimumab in patients with metastatic melanoma. N Engl J Med 2010;363(8):711–23.

77. Brahmer JR, Drake CG, Wollner I, et al. Phase I study of single-agent anti-programmed death-1 (MDX-1106) in refractory solid tumors: safety, clinical activity, pharmacodynamics, and immunologic correlates. J Clin Oncol 2010;28(19): 3167–75.

Transoral Endoscopic Surgery
New Surgical Techniques for Oropharyngeal Cancer

Ryan J. Li, MD, Jeremy D. Richmon, MD*

KEYWORDS

- Oropharynx • Oropharyngeal cancer • Transoral robotic surgery
- Transoral laser microsurgery • Tonsil • Tongue base • TORS • TLMS

KEY POINTS

- Surgery of oropharyngeal cancers has evolved from extensive open approaches with significant associated morbidity to minimally invasive approaches through the mouth.
- Transoral laser microsurgery and transoral robotic surgery are 2 different techniques of transoral endoscopic surgery that can achieve complete oncologic tumor resection without cosmetic deformity while optimizing functional rehabilitation.
- An up-front surgical approach allows tailored adjuvant treatment based on a patient's disease burden.
- Long-term side effects associated with chemotherapy and radiation may be reduced or avoided in carefully selected patients undergoing transoral surgical resection.
- Transoral endoscopic surgery will play an increasing role in the treatment of human papillomavirus–associated oropharyngeal cancer as incidence continues to increase.

Key Abbreviations: TRANSORAL ENDOSCOPIC SURGERY	
AESOP	Automated Endoscopic System for Optimal Positioning
NCCN	National Comprehensive Cancer Network
OP	Oropharyngeal
OPSCCa	Oropharyngeal squamous cell carcinoma
PSS-HN	Head and Neck Performance Status Scale
QOL	Quality of life
TES	Transoral endoscopic surgery
TLMS	Transoral laser microsurgery
TORS	Transoral robotic surgery

Funding support: None.
Financial Disclosure: Dr Richmon is a consultant for Intuitive Surgical, Inc.
Department of Otolaryngology–Head and Neck Surgery, Johns Hopkins University, 601 North Caroline Street, JHOC 6th Floor, Baltimore, MD 21287, USA
* Corresponding author.
E-mail address: jrichmo7@jhmi.edu

Otolaryngol Clin N Am 45 (2012) 823–844
doi:10.1016/j.otc.2012.04.006
0030-6665/12/$ – see front matter © 2012 Elsevier Inc. All rights reserved.

HISTORICAL PERSPECTIVES
Surgery

Until the first quarter of the nineteenth century, there were few reports of operations of the head and neck for cancer, other than for the lip and oral tongue. Before the advent of anesthesia, the pain and inability to restrain even the most willing of patients precluded more than simple and rapid excisions of small tumors.

Although the discovery of anesthesia (ether, 1842; nitrous oxide, 1844; chloroform, 1847) rendered invasive procedures more tolerable, these inhalational gases and the cumbersome apparatuses necessary to administer them made manipulation in the mouth and throat and the control of bleeding even more difficult. Even if surgery were successful, there was no method of alimentation other than an oral diet and no antibiotic treatment to control infection. Postoperative care consisted of extended periods of bed rest (4–6 days after a general anesthetic, 48 hours after local anesthesia) because the benefits of early ambulation were not appreciated. High mortality resulted from exhaustion, general sepsis, and hemorrhage.

The limitations imposed by inhalational anesthetics made radiation the favored treatment method for tumors of the pharynx and larynx in the early 1900s. In the mouth, this was sometimes combined with cautery and endothermy excision either soon after the application of interstitial radon or later, when radionecrosis developed. Large wounds developed, were left open, and frequently resulted in bleeding requiring the ligation of one or both carotid arteries, which became one of the most common procedures performed. Postradiation edema with resultant airway obstruction was common in patients treated for pharynx and larynx cancer and led to many emergent tracheotomies.

In the late 1930s and 1940s, several important medical developments led to the advancement of head and neck surgery. The introduction of sulfa drugs and, later, penicillin, greatly reduced infection and the rates of postoperative wound dehiscence and fistula formation. The introduction of intravenous Pentothal anesthesia freed the surgeon from having to contend with large, cumbersome inhalational devices and led to the development of endotracheal tubes. Blood banks made transfusions possible in the event of life-threatening blood loss. The drum dermatome allowed for the harvest of large, split-thickness skin grafts of uniform thickness to cover extensive surface defects in the head and neck. These advances made radical head and neck surgery possible. Where previously the extent of extirpation was limited by such complications as shock, asphyxia, hemorrhage, infection, sepsis, and failure of wound healing, the primary limitation became the preservation of those structures necessary to maintain a patient's life.

New surgical prowess led to the evolution of open surgical approaches to the oropharynx, including the lateral pharyngotomy, anterior pharyngotomy, mandibulotomy, and lingual release. These approaches start from the outside of the neck and move inward toward the mucosa of the upper aerodigestive tract, which can facilitate the identification and preservation of major neurovascular structures. They are frequently performed with an ipsilateral neck dissection and mandibulectomy (ie, Commando procedure). These procedures led to a great improvement in oncologic outcomes for patients with oropharyngeal cancer, but at a significant price. They result in large incisions with significant tissue dissection and distortion, disruption of the native musculature, and violation of the pharyngeal mucosa with resulting compromise in speech, swallow, and airway function. Patients often require temporary or permanent tracheotomies and feeding tubes and may require extensive rehabilitation. It was not until the end of the twentieth century, when technologic developments led to minimally invasive approaches to the upper aerodigestive tract combined with a human papillomavirus (HPV) epidemic, that a new era of oropharyngeal cancer surgery began.

Radiation and Chemotherapy

Although radiation therapy had an integral role in treatment of upper aerodigestive tract cancers in the early 1900s, it was eventually eclipsed as the first-line treatment modality by the advances in anesthesia and surgery mentioned earlier. However, the second half of the twentieth century saw great developments in radiation technology. In the 1970s, computers were introduced into treatment planning and, in combination with new imaging techniques of computed axial tomography, magnetic resonance imaging, and positron emission tomography scans, improvements in accurately targeting and dosing tumors of the head and neck became possible. More recent developments in intensity-modulated and image-guided radiotherapy led to further refinements while limiting toxicity to healthy tissue.

Concurrent advances in chemotherapy with the introduction of taxanes and biotargeted therapies such as cetuximab intensified the effects of radiation. Oncologic outcomes for patients treated nonoperatively eventually rivaled those treated by upfront surgery. However, the side effect profile and complications for traditional, open surgery remained high, whereas that of radiation and chemotherapy became more tolerable. This difference is shown in a meta-analysis by Parsons and colleagues.[1] In a compiled report of 51 retrospective studies including 6400 patients with tonsillar cancer who underwent surgery (with or without radiation) and radiation (with or without neck dissection) at North American academic medical centers, the rates of local control, locoregional control, 5-year survival, and 5-year cause-specific survival were similar between the 2 groups. However, the rates of severe or fatal complications were significantly greater for the up-front surgery group (23%) compared with the radiation groups (6%). Furthermore, the available data on the functional consequences of treatment suggested the superiority of a nonsurgical approach. These data, combined with emerging studies showing the equivalence of combined-modality organ-preservation chemoradiation compared with total laryngectomy for advanced laryngeal cancer,[2] led to a gradual shift in treatment paradigms for oropharyngeal cancer from operative to nonoperative treatment.

Because of the inherent morbidity of surgery and equivalent oncologic outcomes, nonsurgical treatment gained momentum at the end of the twentieth century. Nonetheless, to date, there is insufficient evidence showing a superior treatment response obtained from surgery or radiation with or without chemotherapy. The only randomized, prospective study comparing surgery versus radiation in the management of advanced head and neck cancer is the Radiation Therapy Oncology Group (RTOG) 73-03 trial.[3] A subgroup of 70 patients with oropharyngeal cancer was randomized to receive either preoperative radiation, postoperative radiation, or radiation alone. There was no statistically significant difference in overall survival between these groups, although the study has been criticized for being underpowered. In contrast, a retrospective analysis of the National Cancer database has indicated that up-front surgical treatment of oropharyngeal cancer followed by radiation treatment does afford a survival benefit compared with radiation and chemoradiation alone.[4]

In Hayes Martin's[5] landmark book *Surgery of Head and Neck Tumors* he recalls lamenting in the early 1920s the common belief that radiation therapy would entirely replace surgery in the treatment of cancer. As a resident, he regretted being born too late to ever be able to perform a total laryngectomy. This sentiment resonates with many young otolaryngologists who have completed training in the last 20 years. With the advent of modern chemoradiation, surgery of the oropharynx has been relegated to a salvage undertaking in many institutions. Just as Dr Martin went on to learn the integral role of surgery in laryngeal cancer, we too are realizing the increasing role of primary surgery in the treatment of oropharyngeal cancer with the advancements of minimally invasive surgical approaches.

CURRENT MINIMALLY INVASIVE SURGICAL APPROACHES

Minimally invasive surgery is designed to reduce morbidity and mortality without compromising oncologic outcomes. The ideal minimally invasive approach to the oropharynx is via a transoral approach, thereby limiting tissue dissection, disruption of speech and swallow musculature, minimizing blood loss, avoiding major neurovascular structures, and limiting injury to normal tissue. Transoral approaches to the oropharynx have traditionally been limited to those tumors that can be directly visualized and manipulated with standard instrumentation and lighting. Because of line-of-sight limitations for tumors in the base of the tongue, transoral approaches had been reserved for smaller lesions of the tonsil and palate. However, in the last 20 years, innovation in surg tech has greatly expanded the ability to resect tumors of the oropharynx via a transoral approach (**Table 1**). Transoral laser microsurgery (TLMS) and transoral robotic surgery (TORS) are the principal minimally invasive transoral endoscopic approaches used for the oropharynx to currently.

Table 1
Inclusion and exclusion criteria for consideration of minimally invasive transoral surgery of the oropharynx: the roles of tumor size (T stage) and HPV status in treatment decision making continue to evolve

Inclusion	Exclusion
T1/T2 oropharynx lesions	Involvement of carotid artery, prevertebral fascia, mandible
NO, N1, N2a, N2b neck disease	Distant metastasis
	Patients who will definitively need chemoradiation despite surgical intervention (obvious extracapsular nodal extension, low likelihood of obtaining negative margins at the primary site)
	Extensive unilateral or bilateral soft palate involvement
	Extension of disease into the nasopharynx
	Tonsillar lesions with extension along the posterior pharyngeal wall past the midline
	Deep base of tongue lesions with extension to the contralateral side
	T4 lesions
	Trismus or other anatomic factors precluding transoral access to the oropharynx
Possible Operative Candidates	—
T3 disease	—
Cystic N3 disease	—
HPV-negative oropharynx tumors may best be treated by surgery followed by chemotherapy and radiation, given their poor prognosis	—

TLMS

Technologic advancements in both binocular microscopy and surgical lasers made precise tissue cutting with minimal blood loss possible. In addition, the recognition that tumors in the upper aerodigestive tract need not be removed in continuity with cervical lymph nodes, and that they may be removed piecemeal without resultant tumor dissemination, led to the development of TLMS in the 1960s and 1970s. Since its inception in Europe, where TLMS showed excellent functional and oncologic outcomes for early stage laryngeal cancer,[6,7] its role has expanded to the pharynx and oral cavity. It has since become a well-established technique in the treatment of oropharyngeal tumors, as initially described by Steiner and colleagues[8] in 2003.

A representative operating room setup for TLMS is shown in **Fig. 1**. The basic instruments include a laser delivery device, binocular operating microscope, a mouth gag with tongue retractor or laryngoscope, and microlaryngeal instruments. A 10,600-nm carbon dioxide (CO_2) laser is frequently used. The CO_2 laser beam is absorbed by water at the tissue-laser interface and transformed into thermal energy, which results in precise tissue cutting. The depth of laser penetration is superficial and thereby predictable. By adjusting the focal length of the laser, its ability to cut rather than photocoagulate or ablate tissue can be varied. The laser becomes a versatile tool by further altering the power, spot size, and duration of pulse. The laser has recently become coupled to computer systems that control the shape, size, and pattern of the beam, allowing for precise, reproducible movements.

The laser has traditionally been coupled to the operating microscope. The linear path of the laser from the microscope creates line-of-sight limitations with the inability to see or deploy the laser around curved surfaces. This limitation is particularly challenging for tumors of the base of the tongue, where only the most anterior edge or protrusion of the lesion is visualized and accessible by the laser. Within the last 5 years, fiberoptic delivery systems for CO_2 and other lasers have been developed. Line-of-sight restraints are partially avoided with the fiberoptic lasers and flexible delivery instruments, which allow greater angles of approach to tumor resection.[9] Rather than aiming the laser from the microscope to a distant point within the patient's mouth, the tip of the laser device is placed within the oropharynx and allows greater freedom of movement.

Excellent technical accounts of TLMS surgical approaches to the oropharynx have been discussed elsewhere and are beyond the scope of this article.[8,10] One

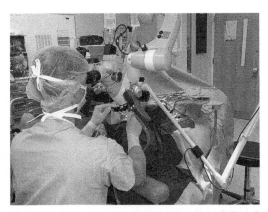

Fig. 1. TLMS operative arrangement. The basic instruments include a laser delivery device, binocular operating microscope, a mouth gag with tongue retractor or laryngoscope, and microlaryngeal instruments.

characteristic particular to TLMS is that line-of-sight limitations, narrow field of vision, and tumor size require that most tumors are removed piecemeal after bisecting the lesion. Although initially anathema to the principles of head and neck surgical oncologists, the oncologic safety of this practice has been substantiated with long-term follow-up showing equivalence to en bloc resections. Both piecemeal and en bloc resections have been described to achieve negative margins with minimal injury to normal tissue.[11–14] Potential disadvantages of TLMS include a steep learning curve and the use of only 1 hand to hold an instrument while the other manipulates the laser.

There are also unique safety concerns to the patient and operating room staff when delivering the intense, focused energy of laser devices. Staff are susceptible to errant laser beams and must wear eye protection. The patient also is at risk of inadvertent burns. Damp towels should cover the eyes and exposed skin of the patient's head and neck, and also reflective surfaces (eg, metallic laryngoscope, suspension bar). A laser endotracheal tube and close communication with anesthesia is mandatory to help prevent the most feared complication of airway fire.

Transoral Robotic Surgery

The first surgical application of a robot was in 1985 when the PUMA 560 placed a needle for brain biopsy by computed tomography guidance. The first robotic system, known as Automated Endoscopic System for Optimal Positioning (AESOP), was approved by the US Food and Drug Administration (FDA) in 1993. It provided a robotically controlled arm to manipulate an endoscope for laparoscopic surgery. This device led to the evolution of the da Vinci Surgical System (Intuitive Surgical, Inc, Sunnyvale, CA), which was FDA approved for abdominal laparoscopic surgery in 2000 and for transoral otolaryngology surgical procedures restricted to T1 and T2 benign and malignant lesions in 2009.

The robot consists of several key components (**Fig. 2**):

- Surgeon console
- Patient-side cart
- Vision system
- Endowrist instruments.

The surgeon console provides a three-dimensional (3D), high-definition image of the operative field and the master controls for the robotic arms and video endoscope. It is positioned at a distance from the patient. The patient-side cart is positioned next to the patient and includes 3 or 4 robotic arms delivering the surgical instruments and video endoscope. This setup is a master-slave system, and surgeon input is required for all robotic movement. The vision system includes a 3D high-definition 0° or 30° endoscope coupled to an image processing tower and monitor for the operating room staff and assisting surgeon. The endowrist instruments are articulating wristed instruments with 7° of freedom in both 8-mm and 5-mm sizes. A typical setup for TORS is shown in **Fig. 3**. The table is rotated 180° from anesthesia. The patient is appropriately relaxed to allow the placement of a mouth gag and suspension. Three of the robotic arms (scope in the center flanked by right and left 5-mm effector arms) are advanced through the mouth. A 0° or 30° scope can be used for tonsil resections and a 30° scope affords optimal visualization of the tongue base. The assisting surgeon sits at the head of the bed and uses an instrument (typically a suction, cautery, retractor, or clip device) in each hand, which allows for 2 surgeons and 4 instruments working at the same time in the oropharynx.

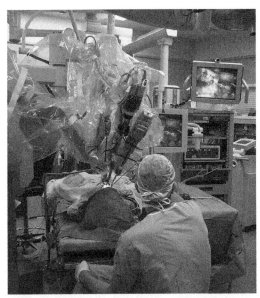

Fig. 2. TORS operative arrangement. The robot consists of several key components: the surgeon console (not shown), the patient-side cart, the vision system, and the endowrist instruments.

TORS provides the surgeon with:

- A 3D, high-definition view of the operative field from the perspective of being inside the mouth of the patient
- A 30° maneuverable scope that affords a wide field of vision, including around the tongue base

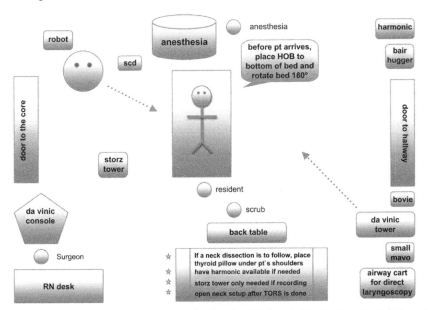

Fig. 3. The operating room arrangement for TORS. HOB, head of bed; pt, patient; RN, registered nurse; SCD, sequential compression device.

- Wristed instruments with tremor-filtration, motion scaling, and 540 degrees of motion to provide precise bimanual tissue manipulation in areas heretofore inaccessible
- Capability of en bloc excision of large oropharyngeal tumors, which some surgeons favor more than TLMS
- No constraints of line-of-sight issues and 1-handed surgery as with TLMS.

Disadvantages include the high cost of the robotic system, logistics of sharing the robot among multiple surgical specialties, need to stage the neck dissection, and training and credentialing requirements. Notable advantages and disadvantages of TORS and TLMS are identified in **Table 2**.

DEVELOPMENT OF TORS

McLeod and Melder[15] were the first to describe using the robot via a transoral approach to biopsy and marsupialize a vallecular cyst in 2005. They also reported their experience setting up the robotic system using porcine and cadaveric models.[16] During the vallecular cyst excision, 2 of the robotic arms were used through a suspended, slotted laryngoscope. Early challenges included a prolonged setup time while attempting to orient the robotic system in relation to the patient. Also in 2006, Hockstein and colleagues[17] from the University of Pennsylvania initiated a series of articles describing the safety and feasibility of TORS from preclinical to clinical experience. These publications elegantly show the rapid evolution of a surgical technology from the laboratory setting to the operating room. This initial success was followed by a TORS phase I trial at the University of Pennsylvania enrolling 27 patients with tonsillar squamous carcinoma; 24 out of 27 were stage III to IV (including 16 T2, 6 T3).[18] Twenty-six of 27 patients were swallowing without needing a gastrostomy tube for supplemental nutrition. This study supported the safety of TORS for tonsillar squamous carcinoma, and provided important momentum for additional studies of TORS for oropharyngeal squamous cell cancer. This work led to a multicenter investigation of TORS showing equivalent or superior oncologic and functional outcomes to open and other transoral surgical approaches, culminating in FDA approval in late 2009.

Table 2	
Advantages and disadvantages of TORS and TLMS	
Advantages	**Disadvantages**
TORS	
3D, high-resolution image	Lack of tactile feedback
Overcomes line-of-sight constraints	Cost of robotic system
Wide field of view	Sharing robot with other services
Bimanual manipulation	Training and credentialing requirements
Tremor-filtration, motion scaling	—
Allows for en bloc resection	—
TLMS	
Ease of startup	Narrow field of view
Precise binocular vision	Single-hand surgery
Ability to differentiate normal from abnormal tissue with laser	Steep learning curve
	Line-of-sight limitations
Ability to reach larynx/hypopharynx	Laser safety issues

Staged Versus Concurrent Neck Dissection

Most patients undergoing TORS receive ipsilateral or bilateral neck dissections. Investigators have favored either a concurrent[19] or a staged[20] neck dissection. Advocates of a concurrent neck dissection note the advantages of:

- A single anesthetic session
- More rapid ultimate recovery and completion of cancer treatment
- Lower costs.

Advocates of a staged procedure allege:

- Less airway edema after TORS if the ipsilateral lymphatics are not disrupted.
- Advantages of waiting on permanent margins from the primary tumor before the neck dissection.
- A greater risk of fistula has also been cited with a concurrent neck dissection.[20] However, Moore and colleagues[19,21,22] recently showed that, despite identifying an oropharyngeal communication in 29% of patients, only 4% went on to develop fistulas.
- Perhaps the greatest driving force of staging the neck dissection is logistics. Performing a concurrent neck dissection effectively occupies the robot for several hours because most facilities have dedicated robotic operating room suites and prohibit the removal of the robot from the room. With robot use approaching saturation at many hospitals, there is growing pressure not to occupy the robot for more time than is necessary.

TORS Postoperative Treatment

The postoperative treatment protocol for patients undergoing TORS ranges from conservative[19,21,22] to more aggressive[23,24] initiation of postoperative feeding. Postoperative treatment at Johns Hopkins Hospital includes:

- 24 hours of intravenous steroids and antibiotics to assist with airway edema, nausea, pain, and decreasing bacterial overgrowth within the open pharyngeal wound.
- Patients admitted for 23-hour observation to the head and neck surgical ward.
- Patients observed overnight in the intensive care unit if they require delayed extubation, are thought to be at significant risk of airway edema, or have a history of obstructive sleep apnea.
- A small-caliber nasogastric tube is placed in all patients prophylactically before emergence from anesthesia.
- Patients are maintained well hydrated with aggressive pain control overnight.
- On the first postoperative morning, a bedside swallow evaluation is performed by a member of the surgical team or speech language pathology. If successful, the nasogastric tube is removed and the patient is initiated on a clear liquid diet and allowed to advance as tolerated. Otherwise, alimentation via tube feeds is begun.
- Patients are usually discharged home on postoperative day 1 with pain medication and a tapering dose of steroids.
- If a neck dissection is done concurrently. the patient is given the option of staying until the drain is removed or going home with drain care instructions.

We have been successful with a rapid return to oral alimentation and short inpatient stays.

ADVANTAGES OF UP-FRONT SURGERY

Perhaps the greatest advantage of up-front transoral endoscopic surgery is the ability to provide pathologic staging information that may determine the intensity of the overall treatment plan. Adjuvant therapy may thereby be tailored to a patient's particular disease burden in contrast with primary radiotherapy, which relies on clinical staging and the inherent pitfalls of overstaging and understaging.

Walvekar and colleagues[25] retrospectively examined the role of primary surgical therapy for early local stage oropharyngeal squamous cell carcinoma (OPSCCa) (T1-2), as well as clinically N1 nodal disease. Conclusions are limited by small sample size (n = 49); however, several interesting findings were reported:

- Postoperative pathologic staging led to upstaging of 7 of 27 (26%) patients who were clinically staged N0, and downstaging of 4 of 19 (21%) patients who were clinically staged N1
- Two of 18 clinically T1 tumors were upstaged to pT2, whereas 11 of 31 clinically T2 tumors were downstaged to pT1
- In summary, the investigators reported that 20 of 49 (40%) patients had adjusted pathologic staging after surgery, with 12 (24%) downstaged.

This information led to withholding of radiation and/or chemotherapy in patients who were downstaged from advanced to early stage. This decision has been supported by various investigators showing a significant reduction in the use of radiation and chemotherapy with an up-front surgical approach.[10,19,21,22,25–30] This may eventually translate into significant overall cost savings as adjuvant treatment is limited and patients return to work sooner. With improvements in transoral endoscopic surgery (TES), surgical, medical, and radiation oncology fields may be equipped to refine OPSCCa staging and make further strides in treatment optimization, respecting both functional and oncologic goals. From an oncologic perspective, the perceived competing roles of TES and nonsurgical modalities are complementary. Accurate surgical staging leads to optimal use of adjuvant therapy.

ONCOLOGIC OUTCOMES FOR OROPHARYNGEAL CANCER TREATED BY TRANSORAL ENDOSCOPIC RESECTION

TLMS and TORS are different surgical techniques that achieve the same common goal: a minimally invasive transoral resection to negative margins. When evaluating functional and oncologic outcomes, we think that these techniques, which respect the basic oncologic tenets, can be collectively grouped as TES. This grouping not only simplifies data interpretation among different studies but it avoids the confusion of having multiple terms that relate more to the surgical tool than to the surgical outcome.

Prospective randomized clinical trials comparing primary TES with nonsurgical treatments for OPSCCa are not available. However, studies examining oncologic outcomes of TES techniques have consistently shown equivalent, if not superior, results to nonoperative treatment protocols.[10] Although TLMS has stood the test of time, there remains controversy about TORS as mature oncologic outcomes data are emerging.

One imperative goal of resection is obtaining negative margins. Machtay and colleagues[31] showed that achievement of negative margins always results in local control. Data from multiple institutions with TORS have positive margin rates in the oropharynx of ~4% compared with 24% to 36% for open resections.[32–34] **Table 3** gives an overview of results from various studies focusing on TLMS and TORS in OPSCCa. Attention is focused on local and regional control, disease-free (recurrence-free) survival, disease-specific survival, and overall survival.[10] Although the data may be criticized as noncontrolled and retrospective, disease-free and overall survival rates greater than 90% for advanced staged disease challenges that of any nonsurgical approach and warrants continued investigation.

HPV-Related Oropharyngeal Cancer

As discussed in elsewhere in this issue, an epidemic of oropharyngeal cancer related to the human papillomavirus is occurring. Although the overall incidence of head and neck cancer is decreasing, recognized cases of HPV-related OPSCCa are increasing. Prior studies cite an increasing proportion of OPSCCa cases related to HPV, perhaps 50% or greater.[35–37] Approximately 80% of all oropharyngeal cancers treated at Johns Hopkins Hospital are HPV related. Both retrospective and prospective studies have shown an improved overall survival in HPV-positive OPSCCa versus HPV-negative related counterparts; an outcome thought to hold true for both surgical and nonsurgical modalities.[35,37–39] Furthermore, patients with oropharyngeal cancer who are HPV positive tend to be younger and healthier than their HPV-negative counterparts. With a greater likelihood of survival and a longer life span over which long-term complications of treatment may manifest and debilitate, the choice of optimal treatment modality becomes even more imperative for these patients. Accordingly, there has been much interest in stratifying treatment of patients with OPSCCa based on HPV status. Currently, the National Comprehensive Cancer Network (NCCN) does not use HPV status to dictate treatment, although it is an active area of clinical research. Active clinical trials for HPV-positive oropharyngeal cancer can be found at http://www.clinicaltrials.gov.

Licitra and colleagues[35] in 2006 reviewed a cohort of 90 patients with OPSCCa treated primarily with surgery and adjuvant radiation when appropriate. Although this study did not specifically focus on transoral surgical approaches, their analysis showed that HPV-positive cancers were associated with improved:

- Overall survival
- Recurrence rates
- Second primary tumor incidence.

Although there remains an absence of level I data comparing surgery with radiation with or without chemotherapy in HPV-positive oropharyngeal cancer, several retrospective reviews of prospectively collected data provide insight into the feasibility of TLMS and TORS in this group.

Rich and colleagues[36] in 2009 sought to identify prognostic factors affecting overall and disease-specific survival in patients with OPSCCa treated with TLMS with or without adjuvant radiation therapy. They reviewed a cohort of 84 patients with advanced stage OPSCCa:

- Seventy-three of these patients had available p16 immunohistochemical testing, of whom 69 (95%) tested positive
- HPV in-situ hybridization testing was positive in 60 (out of 78; 77%) tumors
- p16 status remained a significant predictor of overall survival and disease-specific survival in multivariate analysis.

The investigators concluded that p16 positivity (strongly suggesting HPV infection) predicted better survival outcomes after TLMS with or without radiation therapy, validating transoral surgery as a primary treatment option in HPV-related OPSCCa.[36]

The University of Pennsylvania has also recently reported its experience with primary TORS in the management of OPSCCa, evaluating survival and recurrence

Table 3
A review of oncologic outcomes in studies of transoral surgery oropharyngeal cancer

Reference	Technique	Cancer Site	No. of Patients	AJCC Stage	Adjuvant Treatment	Follow-up (mo)	Disease Control (%)	Disease-free Survival (%)	Disease-specific Survival (%)	Overall Survival (%)	Comments
Henstrom et al,[59] 2009	TLMS	BOT	20	Stage I/II, 1; stage III/IV, 19	RT, 12 (60%); chemotherapy, 4 (20%)	Mean 39.6	83.6 (local), 100 (regional), 94.7 (distant) (2 y)	—	90	90 (2 y), 83.1 (5 y)	4 (20%) did not require adjuvant RT ± chemotherapy
Moore et al,[22] 2009	Transoral NOS	T	102	Stage I/II, 17; stage III/IV, 85	RT, 70 (69%); CRT, 4 (3.9%)	Mean 48	91.8 (local), 97.0 (regional), 91 (distant), (5 y)	—	94	92.2 (2 y), 85 (5 y)	28 (27%) did not require adjuvant RT ± chemotherapy
Steiner et al,[8] 2003	TLMS	BOT	48	Stage I/II, 3; stage III/IV, 45	RT, 11 (23%); CRT, 12 (25%)	Median 47	85 (local) (5 y)	73 (5 y)	—	52 (5 y)	—
Rich et al,[36] 2009	TLMS	46 BOT, 38 T+P	84	Stage III, 13; stage IV, 71	RT, 50 (59%); CRT, 28 (33%)	Median 48.5	94	91 (2 y), 87 (5 y)	96 (2 y), 92 (5 y)	94 (2 y), 88 (5 y)	[a]HPV-association predicted improved overall and disease-specific survival
Camp et al,[60] 2009	TLMS	BOT	71	Stage I/II, 10; stage III/IV, 61	RT, 41 (58%); CRT, 27 (38%)	>24	97% (local), 97% (regional)	90 (2 y)	94 (2 y)	90 (2 y)	—
Grant et al,[61] 2006	TLMS	BOT	59	Stage I/II, 11; stage III/IV, 48	RT 28 (47%)	Mean 31	90 (local) (2 and 5 y), 88 (regional) (2 and 5 y), 97 (distant)	84% (2 and 5 y)	—	—	91 (2 y), 69 (5 y)	—

Study	Approach	Subsites	N	Stage	Adjuvant therapy	Follow-up (mo)	Local/regional control	Survival	Survival	Survival	Comments
Haughey et al,[10] 2011	TLMS	106 BOT, 98 T+P	204	Stage III, 49; stage IV, 155	RT, 117 (58%); CRT, 33 (16%)	Mean 48, median 42	—	85 (2 y), 82 (3 y), 74 (5 y)	91 (2 y), 88 (3 y), 84 (5 y)	89 (2 y), 86 (3 y), 78 (5 y)	[a]HPV surrogate p16+IHC predicted improved survival compared with p16-
White et al,[62] 2010[b]	TORS	77 OP, 2 OC, 10 larynx	89	Stage I/II, 24; stage III/IV, 65	RT, 56 (63%), chemotherapy, 43 (48%)	Median 26	—	86.3 (2 y)	—	—	26 (29%) did not require adjuvant RT ± chemotherapy
Weinstein et al,[63] 2010	TORS	23 BOT, 23 T, 1 P	47	Stage III, 24; stage IV, 23	RT, 13 (27.6%), chemotherapy, 2 (4%), CRT, 27 (57%)	Mean 26.6	98 (local), 96 (regional), 91 (distant)	96 (1 y), 79 (2 y)	98 (1 y), 90 (2 y)	96 (1 y), 82 (2 y)	—
Genden et al,[24] 2011	TORS	11 BOT, 11 T, 4 OP wall, 1 P, 3 other	30	Stage I/II, 8; stage III/IV, 22	—	Median 20.4	91 (local) (1.5 y), 100 (regional)	78 (1.5 y)	—	90 (1.5 y)	—
Cohen et al,[40] 2011	TORS	24 BOT, 23 T, 2 P, 1 posterior wall	50	Stage I/II, 7; stage III/IV, 43	RT, 12 (24%); chemotherapy, 2 (4%); CRT, 27 (54%)	Mean 23–24.8[b]	—	—	97.8 (1 y), 92.6 (2 y)	95.7 (1 y), 80.6 (2 y)	[a]Outcomes did not differ significantly between HPV-related and negative groups

Abbreviations: BOT, base of tongue; CRT, combined chemoradiotherapy; OC, oral cavity; OP, oropharynx; P, soft palate; p16 IHC, immunohistochemical staining for p16 protein overexpression; RT, radiation therapy; T, tonsil; Transoral NOS, not otherwise specified.

[a] HPV-related OPSCCa (24.8), HPV-negative OPSCCa (23.0).

[b] White et al. 2010: 7 patients underwent TORS as salvage for failed primary RT. Excluding these 7 patients, 2-year recurrence-free survival increases to 86.3%.

data in a mixed HPV-positive and HPV-negative group.[40] Of a total of 50 patients with similar stage distribution, in this retrospective review:

- 37 (74%) were HPV positive
- 13 (26%) were HPV negative
- All patients were treated primarily with TORS for base of tongue or tonsillar squamous carcinoma, with adjuvant radiation with or without chemotherapy as dictated by the pathology
- Overall survival was 97.2% at 1-year follow-up for the HPV-positive group
- Overall survival was 90.9% at 1-year follow-up for the HPV-negative group
- Overall survival was 89.5% at 2-year follow-up for the HPV-positive group
- Overall survival was 80.0% at 2-year follow-up for the HPV-negative group
- Disease-specific survival was 97.2% and 100% at 1-year, and 89.5% and 100% at 2-year follow-up.

The investigators concluded that both groups had favorable outcomes with primary TORS with or without adjuvant chemoradiation. Small sample size failed to show a significant difference in outcomes associated with HPV status. Nonetheless, these oncologic outcomes highlight the benefit of up-front TORS in the HPV-positive patients with oropharyngeal cancer.[40]

FUNCTIONAL OUTCOMES OF TES

The goal of any minimally invasive technique is to reduce morbidity while preserving equivalent oncologic results to open techniques. Although overall survival is the most important outcome for patients who have cancer, many patients make decisions regarding treatment based on quality of life (QOL) and functional outcomes. Patients with oropharyngeal squamous carcinoma may have the lowest QOL and functional outcomes.[41–43] This may be caused by the effects of advanced disease and the subsequent treatment affecting speech and swallow function, as well as the psychological effects of loss of function and physical disfigurement.[44–46] As mentioned earlier, nonsurgical approaches to oropharyngeal cancer grew in popularity because of their perceived avoidance of much of the postoperative morbidity of traditional open approaches to the oropharynx. This trend has resulted in nonsurgical treatment of oropharyngeal cancers as standard protocol at many institutions. However, the dogma that lower morbidity is associated with nonsurgical, so-called "organ-preservation" treatment is now being challenged by the new techniques of TES.

- TES avoids a transcervical and transmandibular approach without the resulting disruption of musculature that may affect long-term speech and swallow function
- The defect of a transoral resection is most often left to heal by secondary intention, thereby creating a contracted, sensate, mucosalized surface
- Tracheotomies, gastrostromies, and flap reconstruction are rarely necessary
- Patients are initiated on a liquid or soft diet early, and often are discharged from the hospital after 1 to several nights
- Immediate postoperative complications are significantly fewer than for open, transcervical approaches.

These advantages translate into significant gains in speech and swallow function and ultimately to overall QOL.

Perhaps of greater import to overall QOL and speech/swallow function is the adjuvant treatment delivered after TES:

- The total dose of radiation received to the oropharynx and neck may be the strongest determinant of overall function,[47-49] with chemotherapy exacerbating these effects.[50] Various studies have shown that, with an up-front TES approach, approximately 30% of patients can avoid radiation and chemotherapy. Those patients with negative prognostic pathologic factors requiring radiation receive a lesser total dose if negative margins are achieved.
- A comparative analysis of high-risk postoperative patients with head and neck cancer shows that those patients with positive margins and/or extracapsular nodal spread benefit from adjuvant chemotherapy with radiation.[51-53]

Therefore, in most carefully selected patients, the long-term toxicity of full-dose radiation and chemotherapy may be avoided with an up-front surgical approach.

QOL Outcomes with TORS Plus Adjuvant Therapy

Leonhardt and colleagues[43] showed that, in those patients treated with TORS and tailored adjuvant radiation with or without chemotherapy, the overall QOL and functional status of patients returned to pretreatment levels as measured by the Head and Neck Performance Status Scale (PSS-HN) and Short Form-8 health surveys. Despite treatment affecting the PSS-HN Eating and Diet domains at 6 months, complete recovery occurred by 12 months. The declines at 6 months correspond with the administration of adjuvant radiation, with chemotherapy intensifying these declines. Treatment with TORS alone did not significantly affect swallowing function at 6 months compared with pretreatment measures. This finding highlights the QOL advantages of an up-front transoral surgical approach followed by adjuvant therapy as determined by pathologic risk stratification. A summary of functional outcomes for both TLMS and TORS shows consistently low rates of permanent tracheotomies and feeding tubes (**Table 4**).

QOL for HPV-Positive Versus HPV-Negative Patients with Oropharyngeal Cancer

Although QOL surveys have not yet stratified for patients with HPV-positive versus HPV-negative oropharyngeal cancer, HPV-positive patients might be expected to fare better, not only because they have a greater likelihood of survival but also because they tend to be younger with fewer medical comorbidities,[54,55] which likely translates to an improved ability to rehabilitate speech and swallow function.

Johns Hopkins Outcomes

At Johns Hopkins Hospital, we have shown that excellent oncologic and functional results are attainable on initiation of a TORS program.[56] Functional outcomes from our initial 20 patients showed that all were discharged home on an oral diet with an average hospitalization time of 1.3 days and no tracheotomies performed. We showed that, despite the technical complexities involved with the introduction of a TORS program into a busy academic medical center, excellent functional outcomes can be expected from the start with careful planning.

CONTROVERSIES AND FUTURE DIRECTIONS
Lack of Prospective, Randomized Clinical Trials

To date, a prospective, randomized clinical trial of TES versus radiation with or without chemotherapy has not been performed. This omission leaves a notable absence of level I evidence on which to base treatment recommendations. Furthermore, recruitment of patients for such a trial is likely not feasible today. Without mature data on the oncologic outcomes of patients undergoing TES, there will continue to be skeptics. All

Table 4
A summary of functional outcomes for TLMS and TORS

Reference	Technique	Cancer Site	No. of Patients	Tracheotomy	G-tube Dependence >2 y (%)	Hospitalization (d)	Functional Measures
Holsinger et al,[64] 2005	Transoral without endoscopic assistance	T	191	3.7% temporary, 0 permanent	0	9	—
Steiner et al,[8] 2003	TLMS	BOT	136	0	6	—	Performance status scale, 92% normalcy of diet; 88% understandability of speech
Rich et al,[36] 2009	TLMS	38 T+P, 46 BOT	84	0	3.4	—	81% with FOSS 0–2
Grant et al,[65] 2009	TLMS	28 T, 28 BOT, 14 other	69	16% temporary, 0 permanent	0	3	98% with normal swallow
Camp et al,[60] 2009	TLMS	BOT	71	0 permanent	0	—	UW QOL, 63% patients rated overall QOL as excellent or very good; 98% had minimal or no swallow impairment; 70% had normal speech
Grant et al,[61] 2006	TLMS	BOT	59	37% temporary, 2% permanent	8	4	Preoperative and postoperative median FOSS was 0, preoperative median speech was 0, postoperative speech was 1
Moore et al,[22] 2009	TORS	19 T, 26 BOT	45	31% temporary, 1 patient for 6 mo	18 temporary, 0 long term	3.8	Normal postoperative speech in all patients

Study	Approach	Subsites	No.	Gastrostomy				Comments
Weinstein et al,[18] 2007	TORS	T	27	2 temporary, 0 permanent	1	—	—	All with normal speech
Genden et al,[23] 2009	TORS	7 T, 3 BOT, 2 palate, 6 other	18	0	0	0	1.7	All with normal speech
Iseli et al,[66] 2009	TORS	33 OP, 6 oral, 12 larynx, 3 HP	47	9.3% temporary, 0 permanent	—	17 at 13-m mean follow-up	—	Mean MDADI global score was 3 with overall score of 65 at 2 mo (vs 3.5 and 75, respectively, before surgery)
Weinstein et al,[63] 2010	TORS	23 T, 23 BOT, 1 palate	47	11% temporary, 0 permanent	2.4	—	—	—
Hurtuk et al,[26] 2011	TORS	47 T, 6 BOT, 4 larynx, 5 lingual tonsil, 1 retromolar trigone, 1 parapharynx	64	0	0	0	3d	11 patients required gastrostomy tube placement for dysphagia during adjuvant RT; none required gastrostomy tube placement perioperatively; 4 patients remained gastrostomy tube-dependent at last follow up, up to 5 months after TORS
Richmon et al,[67] 2011	TORS	8 T, 12 BOT	20	0	0	0	1.3	All with normal speech

Abbreviations: FOSS, Functional Outcome Swallowing Scale; MDADI, MD Anderson Dysphagia Inventory; UW, University of Wasington.

clinicians harbor biases regarding which treatment best serves their patients, and most institutions tend to favor either an up-front surgical approach or radiation with or without chemotherapy for patients with oropharyngeal cancer. Patients are therefore geographically randomized to a particular treatment arm. An initial step toward comparing treatment regimens may include cooperative pooling of these multiinstitutional data specifically to study oncologic outcomes.

Variation in Optimal Adjuvant Treatment Regimens

Another point of controversy relates to the optimal adjuvant treatment regimens after TES. Although criteria for adjuvant radiation after resection of squamous cell carcinoma have been proposed,[57,58] there is considerable variation of radiation dosage delivered to low-risk versus high-risk necks after surgery at different institutions. In addition, many radiation oncologists remain unfamiliar with transoral resection techniques and are not comfortable treating oropharyngeal cancer to lower dosages, even when completely resected. Areas of debate include:

- Treatment of retropharyngeal lymph nodes in tonsil cancers
- Treatment of the contralateral neck for lateralized tongue lesions
- Inclusion or shielding of the primary site if completely resected when the neck warrants radiation.

TORS Training and Credentialing

With regards to TORS, there remains considerable controversy in the training and credentialing of surgeons. Currently, Intuitive Surgical, Inc. supports a few dedicated TORS training programs for surgeons in the United States that most hospitals require a surgeon to complete before credentialing. However, there exists a potential conflict of interest if industry controls the training and credentialing process. Is a resident who has been trained in TORS required to complete Intuitive's training program after graduating from residency to be credentialed at another hospital? Will a surgeon who has never performed transoral surgery be equipped to perform TORS after a training course of 2 to 3 days? Various academic societies are attempting to draft training criteria and recommendations for hospital credentialing to standardize the process and free it from industry's influence. At Johns Hopkins Hospital, we have developed a resident training program in TORS that we hope will serve as a model for other residency training programs.[56]

Patient Selection for Surgical Versus Nonsurgical Approaches

Perhaps the most difficult clinical question in assessing a patient with oropharyngeal cancer is which patient would most benefit from a surgical approach as opposed to a nonsurgical approach. This question remains physician and institutionally dependent and is an evolving concept as surgeons become more comfortable removing larger tumors transorally. Without high-level oncologic data showing superiority of 1 treatment modality compared with another, treatment recommendations are driven by functional and QOL outcomes. The anticipated morbidity of a surgical procedure must be balanced with that of radiation with or without chemotherapy. As transoral surgery continues to gain momentum, future studies will help elucidate these challenging issues.

Technologic Evolution in TLMS and TORS

TLMS and TORS are technologically driven procedures that continue to evolve. In the last several years, various fiberoptic laser platforms have been introduced. These flexible lasers have expanded the ability to work around the tongue base and have overcome some of the limitations of line-of-sight lasers. Robotic surgery continues to grow rapidly. The robot was not designed for transoral applications and its design continues to limit the ability to reach areas of the hypopharynx and larynx. Single-port modifications will emerge in the next several years and likely expand the current ability to work in the upper aerodigestive tract. Combining current robotic technology with image-overlay, intraoperative imaging, ultrasonography, optical coherence tomography, and photodynamic therapy holds promise in the near future and will further broaden the ability to treat disease in this difficult-to-access area.

SUMMARY

TES is a minimally invasive, oncologically sound treatment modality with optimal functional outcomes. The recent development of TORS has added momentum to this approach and will likely continue to grow in the future. It is imperative that researchers continue to collect the highest level data possible comparing surgical with nonsurgical options in patients with oropharyngeal cancer to determine optimal treatment recommendations.

REFERENCES

1. Parsons JT, Mendenhall WM, Stringer SP, et al. Squamous cell carcinoma of the oropharynx: surgery, radiation therapy, or both. Cancer 2002;94(11):2967–80.
2. Weber RS, Berkey BA, Forastiere A, et al. Outcome of salvage total laryngectomy following organ preservation therapy: the Radiation Therapy Oncology Group trial 91-11. Arch Otolaryngol Head Neck Surg 2003;129(1):44–9.
3. Kramer S, Gelber RD, Snow JB, et al. Combined radiation therapy and surgery in the management of advanced head and neck cancer: final report of study 73-03 of the Radiation Therapy Oncology Group. Head Neck Surg 1987;10(1): 19–30.
4. Zhen W, Karnell LH, Hoffman HT, et al. The National Cancer Data Base report on squamous cell carcinoma of the base of tongue. Head Neck 2004;26(8):660–74.
5. Martin H. Surgery of head and neck tumors. 1st edition. Philadelphia: Hoeber-Harper; 1957.
6. Steiner W. Results of curative laser microsurgery of laryngeal carcinomas. Am J Otolaryngol 1993;14(2):116–21.
7. Strong MS, Jako GJ. Laser surgery in the larynx. Early clinical experience with continuous CO_2 laser. Ann Otol Rhinol Laryngol 1972;81(6):791–8.
8. Steiner W, Fierek O, Ambrosch P, et al. Transoral laser microsurgery for squamous cell carcinoma of the base of the tongue. Arch Otolaryngol Head Neck Surg 2003;129(1):36–43.
9. Holsinger FC, Prichard CN, Shapira G, et al. Use of the photonic band gap fiber assembly CO_2 laser system in head and neck surgical oncology. Laryngoscope 2006;116(7):1288–90.
10. Haughey BH, Hinni ML, Salassa JR, et al. Transoral laser microsurgery as primary treatment for advanced-stage oropharyngeal cancer: a United States multicenter study. Head Neck 2011;33(12):1683–94.
11. Steiner W, Ambrosch P. Endoscopic laser surgery of the upper aerodigestive tract: with special emphasis on cancer surgery. Stuttgart: Thieme; 2000.
12. Peretti G, Nicolai P, Piazza C, et al. Oncological results of endoscopic resections of Tis and T1 glottic carcinomas by carbon dioxide laser. Ann Otol Rhinol Laryngol 2001;110(9):820–6.

13. Davis RK, Kriskovich MD, Galloway EB 3rd, et al. Endoscopic supraglottic laryngectomy with postoperative irradiation. Ann Otol Rhinol Laryngol 2004;113(2): 132–8.

14. Motta G, Esposito E, Cassiano B, et al. T1-T2-T3 glottic tumors: fifteen years experience with CO_2 laser. Acta Otolaryngol Suppl 1997;527:155–9.

15. McLeod IK, Melder PC. Da Vinci robot-assisted excision of a vallecular cyst: a case report. Ear Nose Throat J 2005;84(3):170–2.

16. McLeod IK, Mair EA, Melder PC. Potential applications of the da Vinci minimally invasive surgical robotic system in otolaryngology. Ear Nose Throat J 2005;84(8): 483–7.

17. Hockstein NG, O'Malley BW Jr, Weinstein GS. Assessment of intraoperative safety in transoral robotic surgery. Laryngoscope 2006;116(2):165–8.

18. Weinstein GS, O'Malley BW Jr, Snyder W, et al. Transoral robotic surgery: radical tonsillectomy. Arch Otolaryngol Head Neck Surg 2007;133(12):1220–6.

19. Moore EJ, Olsen KD, Martin EJ. Concurrent neck dissection and transoral robotic surgery. Laryngoscope 2011;121(3):541–4.

20. Weinstein GS, Quon H, O'Malley BW Jr, et al. Selective neck dissection and de-intensified postoperative radiation and chemotherapy for oropharyngeal cancer: a subset analysis of the University of Pennsylvania transoral robotic surgery trial. Laryngoscope 2010;120(9):1749–55.

21. Moore EJ, Henstrom DK, Olsen KD, et al. Transoral resection of tonsillar squamous cell carcinoma. Laryngoscope 2009;119(3):508–15.

22. Moore EJ, Olsen KD, Kasperbauer JL. Transoral robotic surgery for oropharyngeal squamous cell carcinoma: a prospective study of feasibility and functional outcomes. Laryngoscope 2009;119(11):2156–64.

23. Genden EM, Desai S, Sung CK. Transoral robotic surgery for the management of head and neck cancer: a preliminary experience. Head Neck 2009;31(3):283–9.

24. Genden EM, Park R, Smith C, et al. The role of reconstruction for transoral robotic pharyngectomy and concomitant neck dissection. Arch Otolaryngol Head Neck Surg 2011;137(2):151–6.

25. Walvekar RR, Li RJ, Gooding WE, et al. Role of surgery in limited (T1-2, N0-1) cancers of the oropharynx. Laryngoscope 2008;118(12):2129–34.

26. Hurtuk A, Agrawal A, Old M, et al. Outcomes of transoral robotic surgery: a preliminary clinical experience. Otolaryngol Head Neck Surg 2011;145(2):248–53.

27. Hurtuk A, Teknos T, Ozer E. Robotic-assisted lingual tonsillectomy. Laryngoscope 2011;121(7):1480–2.

28. Hurtuk AM, Marcinow A, Agrawal A, et al. Quality-of-life outcomes in transoral robotic surgery. Otolaryngol Head Neck Surg 2012;146(1):68–73.

29. Weinstein GS, O'Malley BW Jr, Desai SC, et al. Transoral robotic surgery: does the ends justify the means? Curr Opin Otolaryngol Head Neck Surg 2009; 17(2):126–31.

30. Holsinger FC, Sweeney AD, Jantharapattana K, et al. The emergence of endoscopic head and neck surgery. Curr Oncol Rep 2010;12(3):216–22.

31. Machtay M, Moughan J, Trotti A, et al. Factors associated with severe late toxicity after concurrent chemoradiation for locally advanced head and neck cancer: an RTOG analysis. J Clin Oncol 2008;26(21):3582–9.

32. Agrawal A, Wenig BL. Resection of cancer of the tongue base and tonsil via the transhyoid approach. Laryngoscope 2000;110(11):1802–6.

33. Villarreal Renedo PM, Monje Gil F, Junquera Gutiérrez LM, et al. Treatment of oral and oropharyngeal epidermoid carcinomas by means of CO_2 laser. Med Oral 2004;9(2):172–5, 168–72.

34. Smeele LE, Leemans CR, Langendijk JA, et al. Positive surgical margins in neck dissection specimens in patients with head and neck squamous cell carcinoma and the effect of radiotherapy. Head Neck 2000;22(6):559–63.
35. Licitra L, Perrone F, Bossi P, et al. High-risk human papillomavirus affects prognosis in patients with surgically treated oropharyngeal squamous cell carcinoma. J Clin Oncol 2006;24(36):5630–6.
36. Rich JT, Milov S, Lewis JS Jr, et al. Transoral laser microsurgery (TLM) +/- adjuvant therapy for advanced stage oropharyngeal cancer: outcomes and prognostic factors. Laryngoscope 2009;119(9):1709–19.
37. Fakhry C, Westra WH, Li S, et al. Improved survival of patients with human papillomavirus-positive head and neck squamous cell carcinoma in a prospective clinical trial. J Natl Cancer Inst 2008;100(4):261–9.
38. Gillison M. HPV and its effect on head and neck cancer prognosis. Clin Adv Hematol Oncol 2010;8(10):680–2.
39. Gillison ML. HPV and prognosis for patients with oropharynx cancer. Eur J Cancer 2009;45(Suppl 1):383–5.
40. Cohen MA, Weinstein GS, O'Malley BW Jr, et al. Transoral robotic surgery and human papillomavirus status: oncologic results. Head Neck 2011;33(4): 573–80.
41. Bjordal K, Ahlner-Elmqvist M, Hammerlid E, et al. A prospective study of quality of life in head and neck cancer patients. Part II: longitudinal data. Laryngoscope 2001;111(8):1440–52.
42. Hammerlid E, Taft C. Health-related quality of life in long-term head and neck cancer survivors: a comparison with general population norms. Br J Cancer 2001;84(2):149–56.
43. Leonhardt FD, Quon H, Abrahão M, et al. Transoral robotic surgery for oropharyngeal carcinoma and its impact on patient-reported quality of life and function. Head Neck 2012;34(2):146–54.
44. Colangelo LA, Logemann JA, Pauloski BR, et al. T stage and functional outcome in oral and oropharyngeal cancer patients. Head Neck 1996;18(3):259–68.
45. Rogers SN, Lowe D, Fisher SE, et al. Health-related quality of life and clinical function after primary surgery for oral cancer. Br J Oral Maxillofac Surg 2002; 40(1):11–8.
46. Seikaly H, Rieger J, Wolfaardt J, et al. Functional outcomes after primary oropharyngeal cancer resection and reconstruction with the radial forearm free flap. Laryngoscope 2003;113(5):897–904.
47. Sher DJ, Haddad RI, Norris CM Jr, et al. Efficacy and toxicity of reirradiation using intensity-modulated radiotherapy for recurrent or second primary head and neck cancer. Cancer 2010;116(20):4761–8.
48. Dornfeld K, Simmons JR, Karnell L, et al. Radiation doses to structures within and adjacent to the larynx are correlated with long-term diet- and speech-related quality of life. Int J Radiat Oncol Biol Phys 2007;68(3):750–7.
49. Eisbruch A, Schwartz M, Rasch C, et al. Dysphagia and aspiration after chemoradiotherapy for head-and-neck cancer: which anatomic structures are affected and can they be spared by IMRT? Int J Radiat Oncol Biol Phys 2004;60(5): 1425–39.
50. Henk JM. Controlled trials of synchronous chemotherapy with radiotherapy in head and neck cancer: overview of radiation morbidity. Clin Oncol (R Coll Radiol) 1997;9(5):308–12.
51. Bernier J, Cooper JS. Chemoradiation after surgery for high-risk head and neck cancer patients: how strong is the evidence? Oncologist 2005;10(3):215–24.

52. Bernier J, Cooper JS, Pajak TF, et al. Defining risk levels in locally advanced head and neck cancers: a comparative analysis of concurrent postoperative radiation plus chemotherapy trials of the EORTC (#22931) and RTOG (# 9501). Head Neck 2005;27(10):843–50.

53. Bernier J, Pfister DG, Cooper JS. Adjuvant chemo- and radiotherapy for poor prognosis head and neck squamous cell carcinomas. Crit Rev Oncol Hematol 2005;56(3):353–64.

54. Gillison ML, Koch WM, Capone RB, et al. Evidence for a causal association between human papillomavirus and a subset of head and neck cancers. J Natl Cancer Inst 2000;92(9):709–20.

55. Ringstrom E, Peters E, Hasegawa M, et al. Human papillomavirus type 16 and squamous cell carcinoma of the head and neck. Clin Cancer Res 2002;8(10): 3187–92.

56. Richmon JD, Agrawal N, Pattani KM. Implementation of a TORS program in an academic medical center. Laryngoscope 2011;121(11):2344–8.

57. Salama JK, Saba N, Quon H, et al. ACR Appropriateness Criteria®. Adjuvant therapy for resected squamous cell carcinoma of the head and neck. Oral Oncol 2011;47(7):554–9.

58. Quon H, O'Malley BW Jr, Weinstein GS. Postoperative adjuvant therapy after transoral robotic resection for oropharyngeal carcinomas: rationale and current treatment approach. ORL J Otorhinolaryngol Relat Spec 2011;73(3):121–30.

59. Henstrom DK, Moore EJ, Olsen KD, et al. Transoral resection for squamous cell carcinoma of the base of tongue. Arch Otolaryngol Head Neck Surg 2009; 135(12):1231–8.

60. Camp AA, Fundakowski C, Petruzzelli GJ, et al. Functional and oncologic results following transoral laser microsurgical excision of base of tongue carcinoma. Otolaryngol Head Neck Surg 2009;141(1):66–9.

61. Grant DG, Salassa Jr, Hinni ML, et al. Carcinoma of the tongue base treated by transoral laser microsurgery, part one: untreated tumors, a prospective analysis of oncologic and functional outcomes. Laryngoscope 2006;116(12):2150–5.

62. White HN, Moore EJ, Rosenthal EL, et al. Transoral robotic-assisted surgery for head and neck squamous cell carcinoma: one- and 2-year survival analysis. Arch Otolaryngol Head Neck Surg 2010;136(12):1248–52.

63. Weinstein GS, O'Malley BW Jr, Cohen MA, et al. Transoral robotic surgery for advanced oropharyngeal carcinoma. Arch Otolaryngol Head Neck Surg 2010; 136(11):1079–85.

64. Holsinger FC, McWhorter AJ, Menard M, et al. Transoral lateral oropharyngec-tomy for squamous cell carcinoma of the tonsillar region: I. Technique, complica-tions, and functional results. Arch Otolaryngol Head Neck Surg 2005;131(7): 583–91.

65. Grant DG, Hinni Ml, Salassa JR, et al. Oropharyngeal cancer: a case for single modality treatment with transoral laser microsurgery. Arch Otolaryngol Head Neck Surg 2009;135(12):1225–30.

66. Iseli TA, Kulbersh BD, Iseli CE, et al. Functional outcomes after transoral robotic surgery for head and neck cancer. Otolaryngol Head Neck Surg 2009;141(2): 166–71.

67. Richmon JD, Agrawal N, Pattani KM. Implementation of a TORS program in an academic medical center. Laryngoscope 2011;121(11):2344–8.

Treatment Deintensification Strategies for HPV-Associated Head and Neck Carcinomas

Harry Quon, MD, MS[a,b,c],*, Jeremy D. Richmon, MD[b]

KEYWORDS

- HPV-associated head and neck carcinoma • Radiotherapy
- Treatment deintensfication • Late swallowing complications • De-intensification
- Treatment complications

KEY POINTS

- Radiotherapy treatment intensification strategies can improve local-regional control of head and neck squamous cell carcinoma but with an increased risk of late swallowing dysfunction.
- Radiotherapy-related risk factors include the dose intensity of the radiotherapy, especially with accelerated radiotherapy schedules and schedules delivering a large dose per fraction to large volumes of the pharynx.
- Concurrent chemotherapy can also increase the risk of late swallowing dysfunction.
- Several deintensification strategies remain the subject of ongoing investigations.
- Selected clinical presentations in which transoral surgical approaches can be safely used offer the potential to evaluate the patient's pathological risk with regard to the dose and volume of radiation that is administered along with the use of concurrent chemotherapy.

INTRODUCTION

Management approaches for oropharyngeal squamous cell carcinoma (OPSCC) historically used transcervical and mandibulotomy surgical techniques that emphasized the need to achieve local-regional disease control. This came at the expense of competing goals such as the preservation of swallow and laryngeal function. The impact of these

Disclosure: Consultant, Intuitive Surgical (HQ and JR).
Conflict of interest: None.
[a] Department of Radiation Oncology and Molecular Radiation Sciences, Johns Hopkins University School of Medicine, 401 North Broadway, Suite 1440, Baltimore, MD 21231-2410, USA; [b] Department of Otolaryngology–Head and Neck Surgery, Johns Hopkins University School of Medicine, Baltimore, MD 21231-2410, USA; [c] Department of Oncology, Johns Hopkins University School of Medicine, Baltimore, MD 21231-2410, USA
* Corresponding author. Department of Radiation Oncology and Molecular Radiation Sciences, Johns Hopkins University School of Medicine, 401 North Broadway, Suite 1440, Baltimore, MD 21231-2410.
E-mail address: hquon2@jhmi.edu

Abbreviations: Treatment De-Intensification Strategies for HPV-Associated Head and Neck Carcinomas	
3D-CRT	3D-conformal radiation therapy
EGFR	Epidermal growth factor receptor
EORTC	European Organisation for Research and Treatment of Cancer
HNSCC	Head and neck squamous cell carcinoma
IMRT	Intensity modulated radiotherapy
MDADI	MD Anderson Dysphagia Inventory
OPSCC	Oropharyngeal squamous cell carcinomas
PEG	Percutaneous endoscopic gastrostomy
PRO	Patient-reported outcome
PSS	Performance Status Scale
RTOG	Radiation therapy oncology group
SCM	Sternocleidomastoid
SIB	Simultaneous-in field boost
TORS	Transoral robotic surgery
TLM	Transoral laser microsurgery

functional deficits led many clinicians and investigators to question whether non-surgical treatment alternatives could reduce the functional impact and the overall morbidity involved with classic open en bloc resections while maintaining equivalent oncologic results.[1] As such, the past 30 years has focused on the intensification of non-surgical management strategies for both resectable and unresectable clinical stage III/IV head and neck squamous cell carcinoma (HNSCC). While these efforts have improved the oncologic efficacy of radiotherapy,[2,3] these efforts have largely been predicated on the assumption that preservation of anatomic "structure" would be sufficient for functional integrity. Moreover, the inclusion of heterogeneous stage III/IV cancers has raised questions regarding the generalizability of the survival benefits across various T-stage and N-stage presentations and across the different head and neck subsites.

It is now clear that the high-dose chemotherapy and altered radiotherapy fractionation strategies, which contributed to improvements in survival rates, are also associated with an increased risk of developing late swallowing complications.[4–7] In recent years, the significance of this finding is underscored by the favorable prognosis that has been consistently observed in OPSCC associated with the human papillomavirus (HPV) (as defined by various techniques[8–10]). Such patients are typically younger with fewer competing co-morbidities and, hence, more likely to experience survivorship issues from current treatment approaches. With a diagnosis of head and neck cancer at a younger age and increased survival rates, the development of late swallowing complications becomes significant and is most likely to contribute to poor quality of life.[11] For these reasons, it is of paramount importance to understand the current risk factors that contribute to late swallowing complications and to determine the best strategies for future investigation. These considerations become especially important because efforts are underway to change current treatment paradigms, especially in HPV-associated OPSCC, to reduce the risk of late swallowing complications.

WHAT ARE THE RISK FACTORS FOR LATE SWALLOWING COMPLICATIONS?

In recent years, several large analyses have examined which factors independently contribute to an increased risk of developing late swallowing complications.[4–7,12–14] In general, the endpoints reported for late swallowing complications or dysfunction have been heterogeneous with most of the reports incorporating some measure of percutaneous endoscopic gastrostomy (PEG)-tube dependency. Other measures have included the presence of aspiration (asymptomatic or symptomatic), assessment by speech language pathology, and/or various patient-reported quality of life instruments. At this time, there is little consensus on how late swallowing complications should be defined.

Fig. 1 summarizes risk factors for late swallowing complications and highlights those factors that may be amenable to potential therapeutic modification. Several factors are not amenable to risk reduction but should be recognized as factors contributing to the development of late swallowing complications, such as

- Patient age[5,15]
- Pretreatment swallowing dysfunction due to the tumor[14,16]
- Tumor location.[5–7,16]

These studies reflect both the use of nonconformal radiotherapy techniques[4–6] and in recent years, the use of modern conformal treatment approaches such as intensity-modulated radiotherapy (IMRT).[5,6]

It is clear from these independent analyses that the very strategies that were used to intensify the treatment for HNSCC, such as radiotherapy dose intensification and concurrent chemotherapy, also deleteriously injure the surrounding normal tissues involved with swallowing. The volume of normal tissue that is irradiated also seems to be a consistent and important risk factor that has been observed in several analyses:

- Directly, when the length of the irradiated field is considered[17,18]
- Indirectly, when the T-stage[4–6,12] is considered
- Whether ipsilateral or bilateral necks[6] are irradiated.

Several analyses did not have sufficient patients irradiated to only one side of the neck for the latter to be analyzed.[4,5] In fact, Langendijk and colleagues[6] observed that both advanced T-stage and the irradiation of bilateral necks were independent factors in multivariate analysis. This finding suggests that advanced T-stage may be increasing the risk of swallowing injury beyond its influence of increasing the irradiated volume. Increased T-stage definitions reflect more than the increasing size of the primary tumor, but deep tumor infiltration of the surrounding normal tissues which can result in destruction and altered function of the normal tissues.

Late swallowing complications are generally believed to result from[19,20]

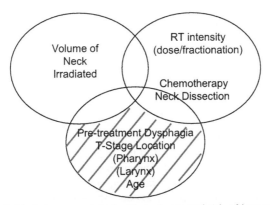

Fig. 1. Summary of risk factors associated with an increased risk of late swallowing complications following radiotherapy for head and neck carcinomas. Potentially modifiable risk factors are distinguished from risk factors, such as the tumor location and patient age, that cannot be therapeutically modified (*diagonal lines*) to reduce the risk of late swallowing complications.

- Direct and fibroproliferative-mediated injury to the neuromuscular units that contribute to both sensation and motor functions involved with swallowing
- Development of chronic inflammation, a consistent observation, and likely to contribute to the underlying mechanism of injury that is an active area of investigation
- Injury to the secretory glands that provide lubrication of the food bolus that can contribute to complaints of dysphagia without any objective evidence of dysmobility.

Radiotherapy as a Risk Factor

Insight into the potential mechanism of late swallowing complications comes from several imaging and retrospective analyses of the dosimetry delivered to various swallowing structures including the pharyngeal constrictor muscles.

Concurrent radiation analysis

In a prospective pilot analysis of 12 patients with HNSCC of the pharyngeal axis treated with concurrent chemoradiation, Popovtzer and colleagues[21] performed MRI of the pharyngeal constrictors at baseline and at 3 months after radiotherapy. These investigators demonstrated

- Significant increase in the T2-weighted signals and thickness of the pharyngeal constrictor muscles that received mean doses greater than 50 Gy compared with mean doses less than 50 Gy[21]
- No significant differences in T1-weighted signals were noted, suggesting that the development of inflammation is dose related
- As a control, analysis of changes in the sternocleidomastoid (SCM) muscles demonstrated a modest increase in T2-weighted signals at 3 months that was not significantly different when partitioned at the mean dose of 50 Gy
- At 3 months, the thickness of the SCM muscles decreased significantly, whereas the thickness in the pharyngeal constrictors increased even for patients receiving less than 50 Gy.

As T2-weighted changes reflect tissue inflammation, these investigators hypothesized that the findings in the pharyngeal constrictors were a consequence of persistent treatment-related acute mucositis. Two patients were noted to be PEG-tube dependent at 3 months, both with elevated T2-weighted signals and thickness in the pharyngeal constrictors. Consistent with this interpretation, Dornfeld and colleagues[22] demonstrated ongoing inflammation (as measured by fluorodeoxyglucose-PET activity) at 12 months postradiotherapy that correlated with late swallowing dysfunction and impaired quality-of-life measures.

The findings by Popovtzer and colleagues[21] suggest that mean doses greater than 50 Gy may be associated with an increased risk of late swallowing complications mediated in part by persistent inflammation. This dose threshold is also suggested in several retrospective studies that have correlated the radiotherapy dose administered to the pharyngeal constrictor muscles and to the supraglottic-endolaryngeal structures and the subsequent development of late swallowing complications.[12,15,23–26] These retrospective studies have demonstrated that exceeding mean doses of 50 to 60 Gy delivered to these structures is associated with an increased risk of swallowing complications.[27]

3D-conformal radiation therapy and IMRT

Characterizing the dose-effect relationship becomes important if, in fact, a dose threshold does exist. The report by Levendag and colleagues[24] offers the greatest insight into the nature of this dose-effect relationship because a wide spectrum of dose delivered to the swallowing muscles was analyzed due to the incorporation of a brachytherapy implant in the management plan. A total of 81 subjects with oropharyngeal carcinomas were treated with either 3D-conformal radiation therapy (3D-CRT) or IMRT, with 53% of subjects also receiving a planned brachytherapy boost. These investigators analyzed

- For RTOG grade 3 toxicities: severe dysphagia requiring enteral support
- For ROTG grade 4 toxicities: complete obstruction, ulceration, perforation, or fistula formation of the esophagus
- And in 64 subjects who were alive and free of disease recurrence: various patient-reported outcome (PRO) measures. These investigators sought to determine the relationship between these endpoints and the dose delivered to the swallowing organs.

The mean doses to various swallowing muscles and structures were calculated based on a summation of dose delivered from brachytherapy and external beam radiotherapy (**Fig. 2**).

With a mean follow-up of 18 months (2–34 months) for IMRT-treated subjects and 46 months (2–72 months) for 3D-CRT–treated subjects, Levendag and colleagues[24] reported a 23% rate of late RTOG grade 3 or 4 dysphagia with a significant association between this late toxicity and the mean dose delivered to the superior (P = .002), middle (P = .003), and inferior (P = .006) constrictor muscles. A threshold dose of 55 Gy (mean) to the superior constrictor muscles for developing late RTOG grade 3 or 4 dysphagia was demonstrated. This risk of dysphagia appeared to increase linearly with increasing dose beyond 55 Gy (see **Fig. 2**). Supporting the notion that a threshold dose effect for the pathogenesis of late swallowing complications may exist.

Gokhale and colleagues[12] observed a similar and significant difference in the risk of late swallowing complications (as defined by the use of PEG tubes for more than 6

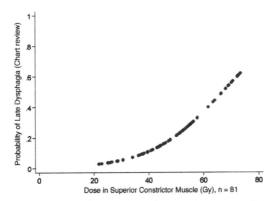

Fig. 2. Significant dose-effect relationship between the mean dose to the superior constrictor muscle and the risk of RTOG grade 3 or 4 dysphagia (P = .002). The probability of late RTOG grade 3 or 4 dysphagia increased significantly with dose, with a suggested threshold dose of 55 Gy and the risk of dysphagia increasing approximately 19% for every additional 10 Gy. (*From* Levendag PC, Teguh DN, Voet P, et al. Dysphagia disorders in patients with cancer of the oropharynx are significantly affected by the radiation therapy dose to the superior and middle constrictor muscle: a dose-effect relationship. Radiother Oncol 2007;85(1):64–73; with permission.)

months) when comparing patients who received 70 Gy versus 60 Gy to the pharyngeal constrictors (**Fig. 3**).

Levendag and colleagues[24] further reported on the results of PROs obtained post-treatment in 88% of subjects without disease relapse. PROs analyzed included the European Organisation for Research and Treatment of Cancer (EORTC) core Quality of Life Questionnaire (QLQ) Core 30 (C30) and the EORTC QLQ-Head and Neck 35 (HN35) swallowing scale. Functional assessment was also analyzed using the observer-reported List Performance Status Scale (PSS) and the patient-reported M.D. Anderson Dysphagia Inventory (MDADI). Although not specified, it appeared that the PROs were obtained at a minimum of 12 months following completion of radiotherapy. Levendag and colleagues[24] clustered the scores in these PROs to derive surrogate grade 3 or 4 toxicity rates and found similar complication rates to the retrospective chart review assessments for RTOG grade 3 or 4 dysphagia:

- HN35: 7–18%
- PSS: 2–30%
- MDADI: 21–32%.

More significantly, dose correlations were also observed with these patient-reported measures of dysphagia offering additional validation of a dose-effect relationship (**Fig. 4**).

Nonconformal radiation therapy

Further validation of a threshold dose for developing dysphagia has also been suggested in the setting of a randomized phase III study of postoperative radiotherapy dose intensification. All subjects were irradiated with a nonconformal technique and would have resulted in most of the pharyngeal constrictor muscles being irradiated. With a median follow-up of 59 months (22–83 months), Ang and colleagues[28] observed

- A late grade 3 or 4 dysphagia rate of 13%–16% in patients receiving 63 Gy post-operatively (without concurrent chemotherapy)

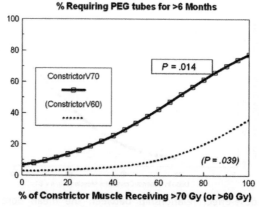

Fig. 3. The risk of late swallowing complications in patients receiving 70 Gy versus 60 Gy to the pharyngeal constrictors. Patients receiving 70 Gy to the pharyngeal constrictors was an independent significant risk factor in logistic multivariate regression analysis for the risk of developing late swallowing complications (defined as requiring a PEG tube >6 months). (*From* Gokhale AS, McLaughlin BT, Flickinger JC, et al. Clinical and dosimetric factors associated with a prolonged feeding tube requirement in patients treated with chemoradiotherapy (CRT) for head and neck cancers. Ann Oncol 2010;21(1):145–51; with permission.)

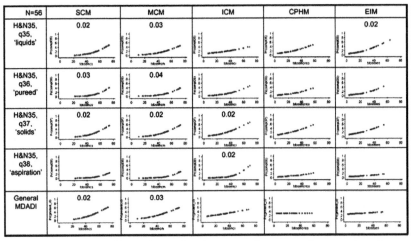

N=56	SCM	MCM	ICM	CPHM	EIM
H&N35, q35, 'liquids'	0.02	0.03			0.02
H&N35, q36, 'pureed'	0.03	0.04			
H&N35, q37, 'solids'	0.02	0.02	0.02		
H&N35, q38, 'aspiration'			0.02		
General MDADI	0.02	0.03			

Fig. 4. Significant dose-effect relationship between the mean dose to the pharyngeal constrictor muscles and the risk of dysphagia as measured by various PRO questionnaires. Summary of the interrelationship between the radiotherapy dose delivered and the risk of various swallowing difficulties as measured by the EORTC QLQ HN35 swallowing scale and the MDADI, distinguished by specific swallowing structures. CPHM, cricopharyngeus muscle; EIM, esophageal inlet; ICM, inferior constrictor muscle; MCM, middle constrictor muscle; SCM, superior constrictor muscle. (*From* Levendag PC, Teguh DN, Voet P, et al. Dysphagia disorders in patients with cancer of the oropharynx are significantly affected by the radiation therapy dose to the superior and middle constrictor muscle: a dose-effect relationship. Radiother Oncol 2007;85(1):64–73; with permission.)

compared with..

- Late grade 3 or 4 dysphagia rate of 4% when 57.6 Gy was delivered.

This study is noteworthy, not only for the randomized prospective nature of the study design, but that patients were treated without concurrent chemotherapy.

Radiotherapy intensification

Radiotherapy intensification using accelerated fractionation schedules with non-conformal radiation techniques has been shown to be a significant risk factor for late swallowing complications in multivariate[6] and univariate analyses.[5,29] A similar inverse correlation between the overall treatment time and the severity of acute mucositis[18] and the risk of late swallowing complications have been reported.[18,30] This risk seems to be also related to the daily dose of radiotherapy, total radiotherapy dose delivered at the end of treatment,[29] and the severity of acute mucositis.[18,31] These observations offer a cautionary lesson on more modern strategies to accelerate the radiotherapy using simultaneous-in field boost (SIB) IMRT strategies.

In fact, similar correlations between SIB-IMRT large daily dose per fractions administered to a large mucosal volume have been observed to cause:

- Unacceptable acute mucositis
- Increased acute dysphagia
- Delayed mucositis healing.

In a phase I dose-escalation study of SIB-IMRT alone, Lauve and colleagues[32] demonstrated acute dose-limiting mucosal toxicities with daily fractions of 2.46 Gy, leading these investigators to conclude that the maximum-tolerated dose was 2.36 Gy. Late toxicities were also reported with grade 3 dysphagia and grade 4 mucosal toxicities seen at 2.36 Gy, suggesting that, in fact, the optimal dose per fraction may be lower.

Bhide and colleagues[18] also performed a phase I dose-escalation SIB-IMRT with concurrent chemotherapy and demonstrated:

- A significant increase in the rate of grade 3 dysphagia with daily fractions of 2.4 Gy compared with 2.25 Gy or less
- A correlation between the length of the radiation field treated to doses of 50 Gy or greater with the risk of grade 3 dysphagia
- A correlation between the duration of grade 3 mucositis (longer than 12 weeks) and the risk of developing late dysphagia at 6 months.

Radiation to ipsilateral neck

Most OPSCC patients typically receive radiation to the primary site and bilateral cervical necks due to the risks of bilateral lymphatic metastases. However, when patients receive radiation to the primary and only the ipsilateral neck, Langendijk and colleagues[6] noted that the risk of late swallowing complications is significantly reduced, even when T-stage was introduced into the multivariate analysis. Similar observations were reported by Frowen and colleagues[7] who demonstrated that irradiation of only the ipsilateral neck significantly reduced the risk of late dysphagia with liquids as evaluated by videofluoroscopy. Consistent with the adverse influence of the high dose irradiated tumor volume was the observation that the length of the nonconformal fields also directly correlated with the risk of swallowing dysfunction at 3 months and a trend at 6 months.[7] Not surprising are similar direct correlations between the length of nonconformal radiation fields and the severity of the acute mucositis and the requirement for PEG support,[17,33] reaffirming that late swallowing complications can arise as a consequence of severe acute mucositis.

In summary, several lines of evidence support the conclusion that the radiotherapy dose and the volume of the pharynx that is irradiated can influence the risk of developing late swallowing complications—increasing when a large volume of the pharynx is irradiated with mean pharyngeal constrictor doses greater than 50 to 60 Gy, as is the case with definitive bilateral neck radiation for oropharyngeal carcinomas. Whether or not specific swallowing regions of the pharynx (such as the inferior constrictor muscles) are more sensitive to radiation-induced injury is not clear at this time. What is clear is that the severity of the acute mucosal injury is correlated with the risk of persistent mucosal inflammation and a potential consequential risk of late swallowing complications. At this time, the exact nature of the dose-volume relationship for late swallowing complications has not been clearly delineated. When considering the mean dose to the irradiated constrictor muscles, there may indeed be a threshold dose for the risk of developing late swallowing complications. Beyond this threshold dose, the risk may increase significantly.

Chemotherapy as a Risk Factor

Concurrent chemotherapy can significantly and independently increase the risk for late swallowing complications. Most of the evidence to date comes in the setting in which high doses such as 70 Gy are planned.[5,6] Multivariate analyses in which a sufficient number of subjects were treated with and without concurrent chemotherapy have demonstrated hazard ratios ranging from 2.6 to 9.[5,6] Whether or not the influence of concurrent chemotherapy is different at lower planned radiotherapy doses to the pharynx is not clear at this time. However, the analysis by Caudell and colleagues[5] demonstrated that when concurrent chemotherapy was modeled with radiotherapy doses less than or greater than 70.4 Gy, the administration of concurrent chemotherapy was not only independently significant but was associated with a ninefold risk in contrast to a nonsignificant influence of the radiotherapy dose partitioned at 70.4 Gy.

The risk of late swallowing complications has not been found to be significantly different between platinum alone and platinum combination chemotherapy regimens, though this observation may be limited by a lack of statistical power in its analysis.[5] It is also not clear if alternative schedules of cisplatin administration, such as weekly low-dose cisplatin, can reduce this risk. In a randomized trial of low-dose weekly cisplatin (20 mg/m^2) with radiotherapy compared with radiotherapy alone, the administration of weekly cisplatin increased the risk of late esophageal (9% vs 3%, $P = .03$) and laryngeal (11% vs 4%, $P = .05$) toxicities when compared with radiotherapy alone.[34] Interestingly, no evidence of tumor radiosensitization was seen.

An alternative radiosensitizing option has been the weekly administration of the epidermal growth factor receptor–binding monoclonal antibody, cetuximab. The results of a large randomized study of concurrent cetuximab and radiotherapy demonstrated that acute mucositis rates may not be significantly increased to that of fractionated radiotherapy alone.[35] This has been interpreted as evidence of potential selective targeting of HNSCC cells. This observation along with the modest spectrum and severity of systemic toxicities has lead to the perception that cetuximab may also have a favorable late toxicity profile. However, the rates of long-term toxicities, especially measures of late swallowing complications, have not been reported, even with long-term follow-up.[36] Hence, the ability to use cetuximab as a strategy to potentiate the effects of radiotherapy while reducing the risk of late swallowing complications is unclear at this time.

Surgery as a Risk Factor

The practice of postradiotherapy prophylactic neck dissections began in response to unsalvageable neck relapses, especially for advanced nodal disease, even when a complete clinical response in the neck was achieved. Although this practice continued even in the era of radiotherapy intensification, the high neck control rates observed may have potentially been confounded by the unrecognized and evolving epidemiology of HPV-associated OPSCC. Moreover, post-chemoradiotherapy neck dissections have recently been associated with an increased risk of late swallowing complications in a recent large analysis of the RTOG database, complicating the risk-benefit assessment of this practice.[4]

Late RTOG grade 3 or 4 laryngeal or pharyngeal dysfunction

Machtay and colleagues[4] performed a case-control analysis comparing 99 subjects with late RTOG grade 3 or 4 laryngeal or pharyngeal dysfunction matched to 131 controls from three previously completed RTOG head and neck phase trials (RTOG 9111, 9703, and 9914). Multivariate analysis demonstrated several factors associated with late laryngeal/pharyngeal dysfunction, including:

- Age (odds ratio [OR] 1.05, $P = .001$)
- Advanced T-stage (OR 3.07, $P = .0036$)
- Larynx or hypopharynx primary site (OR 4.17, $P = .0041$)
- Post-chemoradiation neck dissection (OR 2.39, $P = .018$).

The strength of this analysis is the large study cohort that also included the use of negative matched controls. These results are consistent with consistent with other retrospective reviews.[37,38]

In contrast, Caudell and colleagues did not observe postradiotherapy neck dissections to be significant in their multivariate analysis. Although 69% of the 122 study subjects received concurrent chemotherapy, this analysis may have been underpowered as the number of individuals with late swallowing dysfunction (which was defined as a composite clinical endpoint including the presence of PEG-tube dependency or the presence of aspiration or strictures) who underwent a neck dissection was 12 compared with 35 patients who did not receive a neck dissection. Similarly, the recent retrospective review by Chapuy and colleagues[39] analyzed only patients who received a neck dissection without a cohort of patients without a neck dissection while evaluating for factors that correlated with impaired swallowing.

WHAT ARE POTENTIAL STRATEGIES TO REDUCE TREATMENT-RELATED SWALLOWING COMPLICATIONS?

The current emphasis on reducing the risk of late swallowing complications in the OPSCC patient has primarily centered on the development of new treatment approaches. Past efforts have demonstrated that initiating pretreatment swallowing exercises can improve epiglottic tilt or laryngeal elevation and the range of base of tongue retraction and are important strategies to integrate into current practices.[40,41] At this time, several clinical trials investigating alternative radiotherapy deintensification approaches in the HPV-associated OPSCC patient are actively accruing and results from these studies will not be available for several years (**Table 1**).

Deintensification Clinical Trials for HPV-Associated OPSCC

Several cooperative oncology groups and institutions are actively conducting deintensification clinical trials for HPV-associated OPSCC. These include the evaluation of whether cetuximab can provide selective radiosensitization when compared with radiation and cisplatin while achieving comparable survival with reduced toxicities, especially late swallowing complications (RTOG 1016). The radiotherapy fractionation schedule for both arms uses an accelerated schedule delivering 6 fractions per week to a total dose of 70 Gy over 6 weeks with twice daily radiotherapy with 2 Gy per fraction administered 1 day of the treatment week. Only IMRT is permitted with no SIB prescription. The primary endpoint is overall survival with secondary endpoints of local-regional control rates and acute and late toxicities that include specific focus on quality of life swallowing domains. As described, the assumption that cetuximab can provide selective radiosensitization has largely been inferred from the comparable

Table 1 Current strategies to reduce swallowing complications after treatment of HPV-associated OPSCC			
	Dose Decrease?	Volume Decrease?	Concurrent Sensitizer?
RTOG-1016	−	−	+ (cisplatin vs cetuximab)
ECOG-1308	+	−	+ (cetuximab)
JHU-0988	+	−	−/+ (cisplatin)

acute maximum rates of mucositis between radiotherapy alone and radiotherapy and concurrent cetuximab.[35] Although the results of this large study will be important in deciding if cetuximab can offer a more favorable therapeutic ratio, the use of an accelerated fractionation schedule may confound any selective radiosensitization. In the setting of concurrent chemoradiation with conventional daily fractionation, RTOG 0522 demonstrated that the addition of concurrent cetuximab can increase the rate of grade 3 or 4 mucositis (45% vs 35%, $P = .003$) with no difference in the rate of acute grade 3 or 4 dysphagia (62% vs 66%, $P = .27$). No late toxicities have been reported to date.

Whether induction chemotherapy may allow for a significant reduction in the radiotherapy dose to the primary site (54 Gy with concurrent cetuximab) is being addressed in a prospective and recently completed multi-institutional trial (ECOG 1308). A critical element of this study is that the primary target volume is based on the prechemotherapy primary volume, even if a complete clinical response to the three 21-day cycles of induction cisplatin, paclitaxel, and cetuximab has been achieved. With a complete response at the primary site, the prescribed dose is reduced to 54 Gy from 69.3 Gy for incomplete responses. A response-based prescription approach is also used for metastatic cervical lymph nodes, reducing the dose to 54 Gy for a complete response following induction chemotherapy. This has the potential advantage of further reducing the dose and volume of the pharyngeal constrictors that is irradiated. If the current evidence for a threshold dose-effect is valid, the reduction in the radiotherapy dose even when treating the prechemotherapy volume would be expected to reduce the risk of late swallowing complications.

Finally, whether or not a reduction in the primary site radiotherapy dose without induction chemotherapy can be safely performed is also being prospectively evaluated at the institution level (Johns Hopkins University [JHU]-0988). This trial, which is limited to HPV-associated OPSCC, is prospectively evaluating primary tumor dose reduction from the traditional 70 Gy to 63 Gy with and without concurrent cisplatin (based on nodal indications), seeking to reduce the radiation dose to the surrounding swallowing tissues to minimize the risk of swallowing complications. It is also reducing the dose prescribed to the low-risk but larger planning target volume. Similar efforts are also underway at various other institutions to reduce the adjuvant radiotherapy dose following a transoral robotic surgery (TORS) resection.

Principles to Reduce Risk of Late Swallowing Complications

Outside of the context of a clinical trial, the current standard treatment of 70 Gy to tumor at the primary site should not be modified based on the HPV status. However, when developing a treatment plan, several principles can be applied to reduce the risk of late swallowing complications in the HPV-associated OPSCC patient.

Dose and volume

The first principle is the clear interrelationship between dose and volume to the pharynx and the risk of severe acute mucositis, with persistent posttreatment inflammation and the subsequent risk of late swallowing complications. Although the exact nature of the dose-volume relationship has not been fully characterized, the data to date supports a threshold dose at a mean dose of 55 Gy to the pharyngeal constrictor muscles beyond which the risk may significantly increase. Whether establishing and achieving this as a radiotherapy treatment planning objective can prospectively reduce the risk of late swallowing injury is unclear. However, concerted efforts to reduce the volume of the uninvolved pharynx that is irradiated would seem to be effective.

Unilateral radiation

Frowen and colleagues[7] demonstrated that when the pharynx was unilaterally irradiated through the use of a pharyngeal avoidance volume (aiming to limit the dose to less than 50 Gy), even when bilateral cervical nodal chains were treated, the risk of late swallowing complications as assessed by videofluoroscopy was significantly reduced. Similar observations have been reported by other groups.[42,43] Partial pharyngeal irradiation would seem to especially benefit lateralized oropharyngeal carcinomas, reducing the risk of swallowing complications, especially following TORS that removes the intraluminal tumor mass (**Fig. 5**). This hypothesis is supported by institutional reports demonstrating long-term PEG-tube dependency rates less than 5%.[42,44,45]

Transoral surgical techniques

Transoral surgical techniques, such as TORS and transoral laser microsurgery can facilitate safer tumor exposure and resection of oropharyngeal neoplasms as well as provide pathologic evaluation of the primary tumor and neck nodes, offering several potential advantages. Most significantly, it allows for risk stratification of patients based on objective pathologic criteria to determine the intensity of adjuvant treatment. This allows the physician to distinguish pathologic primary and nodal indications for the use of concurrent chemotherapy. For the primary site, the data supports the use of concurrent chemotherapy only for histologically involved margins at the cut mucosal edge of the tumor specimen.[46,47] It is unclear whether or not concurrent chemotherapy is indicated for suspicious or close (ie, less than 5 mm) margins. For the clinical N1-N2b neck, 30% to 80% of patients may not have pathologic indications (ie, presence of extracapsular extension) for concurrent chemotherapy.[48] Thus, for laterally located OPSCC with N1 to non–bulky N2b disease, in which the probability of achieving a negative margin primary site resection is expected to be high, the use of concurrent chemotherapy can potentially be avoided and the volume of the pharynx that is exposed to high-dose radiation reduced. This is because a major determinant of the pharyngeal volume that is irradiated is related to the presence of an intraluminal mass that is commonly juxtaposed to uninvolved swallowing structures. These structures otherwise will be radiated when the patient is placed in the supine and typically hyperextended neck position that is commonly used for external beam radiotherapy treatment planning.

As the primary oropharyngeal mass approaches the midline, an increasing volume of the circumferential pharyngeal normal tissues becomes exposed to higher does of radiation and has a greater capacity to cause injury. In part, this is due to the use of coplanar arrangements of the beams of radiation all centered on a single isocenter. Although it may be argued that transoral resection allows for lower doses of adjuvant radiotherapy that may be at the threshold of injury (ie, 57.6–63 Gy), the impact of swallowing function with such midline resections is currently undefined. This is further confounded because midline lesions typically require bilateral cervical nodal radiation, increasing the volume of the irradiated midline pharynx. In contrast, lateralized tonsil primary lesions in the setting of N0-1 metastases may confidently be irradiated to only the ipsilateral neck and lateral pharynx because the risk of contralateral nodal metastases is less than 5%.[49] Alternative treatment strategies for midline OPSCC, such as the incorporation of brachytherapy implants for the boost portion of the radiation prescription, may offer some dosimetric advantages. However, the functional impact of these different strategies has not been evaluated to determine the optimal function preserving treatment. In this regard, studies such as E1308 offer an attractive option in the context of a clinical trial because it allows for a significant dose reduction to the midline pharynx.

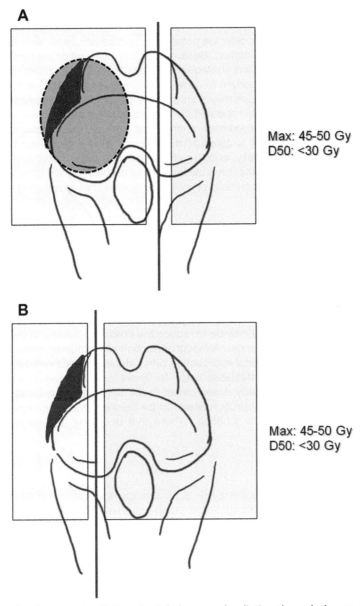

Max: 45-50 Gy
D50: <30 Gy

Max: 45-50 Gy
D50: <30 Gy

Fig. 5. Partial pharyngeal radiation. Partial pharyngeal radiation through the use of a dosimetric avoidance volume demonstrating the ability to reduce the uninvolved side of the pharynx. This strategy can be more favorably applied for lateral oropharyngeal carcinomas (A) especially when only the surgical tonsillar bed requires irradiation (B).

FUTURE DIRECTIONS IN RADIATION DEINTENSIFICATION

Current efforts to deintensify modern radiotherapy are based on the observation that HPV-associated OPSCC not only have a favorable prognosis but that this biomarker seems to predict for a favorable treatment response to radiotherapy. Evaluating and defining potential additional biomarkers will be important to consider as the radiotherapy dose is decreased to identify which patients may require alternative treatment. Refining current therapies that offer the potential to reduce late swallowing function is also an important research direction. Because the selective use of modern transoral surgical techniques already offers strategies to reduce the current treatment morbidity, it will become ever more important to develop techniques to quantify and delineate where these surgical techniques may start to injure patient swallow function in more subtle but potentially clinically meaningful ways. Another future direction will be the development of alternative treatment approaches with nonoverlapping toxicities, including the development of targeted immunotherapy, given the unique biology of HPV-associated OPSCC. Finally, ongoing efforts that advance understanding of the pathophysiology of late radiotherapy-induced normal tissue injury will be important to yield novel therapeutic and potentially prophylactic approaches to reducing late swallowing complications.

SUMMARY

There has been significant progress in understanding the risk factors that contribute to radiation-induced swallowing injury. The most effective strategy to reduce long-term morbidity is to optimize current treatment approaches. Presently, the ability to reduce the prescribed radiotherapy dose, especially in the HPV-positive patient, remains a subject of active clinical investigation and cannot be routinely recommended. A more prudent strategy may be to reduce the irradiated volume of the pharynx and larynx uninvolved with cancer. Although induction chemotherapy may help with this, the use of transoral surgical approaches with pathologic risk stratification of the primary tumor and neck metastases allow for more judicious use of concurrent chemotherapy and radiotherapy doses closer to the suggested threshold for swallowing complications. This approach needs to be balanced with the impact of any surgical resection on swallow function. Where that boundary lays remains to be established.

REFERENCES

1. Khariwala SS, Vivek PP, Lorenz RR, et al. Swallowing outcomes after microvascular head and neck reconstruction: a prospective review of 191 cases. Laryngoscope 2007;117(8):1359–63.
2. Pignon JP, le Maître A, Bourhis J. Meta-analyses of chemotherapy in head and neck cancer (MACH-NC): an update. Int J Radiat Oncol Biol Phys 2007;69 (2 Suppl 1):S112–4.
3. Bourhis J, Overgaard J, Audry H, et al. Hyperfractionated or accelerated radiotherapy in head and neck cancer: a meta-analysis. Lancet 2006;368(9538): 843–54.
4. Machtay M, Moughan J, Trotti A, et al. Factors associated with severe late toxicity after concurrent chemoradiation for locally advanced head and neck cancer: an RTOG analysis. J Clin Oncol 2008;26(21):3582–9.
5. Caudell JJ, Schaner PE, Meredith RF, et al. Factors associated with long-term dysphagia after definitive radiotherapy for locally advanced head-and-neck cancer. Int J Radiat Oncol Biol Phys 2009;73(2):410–5.
6. Langendijk JA, Doornaert P, Rietveld DH, et al. A predictive model for swallowing dysfunction after curative radiotherapy in head and neck cancer. Radiother Oncol 2009;90(2):189–95.

7. Frowen J, Cotton S, Corry J, et al. Impact of demographics, tumor characteristics, and treatment factors on swallowing after (chemo) radiotherapy for head and neck cancer. Head Neck 2010;32(4):513–28.

8. Fakhry C, Westra WH, Li S, et al. Improved survival of patients with human papillomavirus-positive head and neck squamous cell carcinoma in a prospective clinical trial. J Natl Cancer Inst 2008;100(4):261–9.

9. Gillison ML, Harris J, Westra W, et al. Survival outcomes by tumor human papillomavirus (HPV) status in stage III-IV oropharyngeal cancer (OPC) in RTOG 0129. J Clin Oncol 2009;27(15S):6003 [abstract].

10. Worden FP, Hooton J, Lee J, et al. Association of tobacco (T) use with risk of distant metastases (DM), tumor recurrence, and death in patients (pts) with HPV-positive (+) squamous cell cancer of the oropharynx (SCCOP). J Clin Oncol 2009;27(15S):6001 [Abstract].

11. Langendijk JA, Doornaert P, Verdonck-de Leeuw IM, et al. Impact of late treatment-related toxicity on quality of life among patients with head and neck cancer treated with radiotherapy. J Clin Oncol 2008;26(22):3770–6.

12. Gokhale AS, McLaughlin BT, Flickinger JC, et al. Clinical and dosimetric factors associated with a prolonged feeding tube requirement in patients treated with chemoradiotherapy (CRT) for head and neck cancers. Ann Oncol 2010;21(1):145–51.

13. Caudell JJ, Schaner PE, Desmond RA, et al. Dosimetric factors associated with long-term dysphagia after definitive radiotherapy for squamous cell carcinoma of the head and neck. Int J Radiat Oncol Biol Phys 2010;76(2):403–9.

14. Dirix P, Abbeel S, Vanstraelen B, et al. Dysphagia after chemoradiotherapy for head-and-neck squamous cell carcinoma: dose-effect relationships for the swallowing structures. Int J Radiat Oncol Biol Phys 2009;75(2):385–92.

15. O'Meara EA, Machtay M, Moughan J, et al. Associations between radiation doses to pharyngeal regions and severe late toxicity in head and neck cancer patients treated with concurrent chemoradiotherapy–an RTOG analysis. Int J Radiat Oncol Biol Phys 2007;69(Suppl 3):S54–5.

16. Agarwal J, Dutta D, Palwe V, et al. Prospective subjective evaluation of swallowing function and dietary pattern in head and neck cancers treated with concomitant chemo-radiation. J Cancer Res Ther 2010;6(1):15–21.

17. Poulsen MG, Riddle B, Keller J, et al. Predictors of acute grade 4 swallowing toxicity in patients with stages III and IV squamous carcinoma of the head and neck treated with radiotherapy alone. Radiother Oncol 2008;87(2):253–9.

18. Bhide SA, Gulliford S, Fowler J, et al. Characteristics of response of oral and pharyngeal mucosa in patients receiving chemo-IMRT for head and neck cancer using hypofractionated accelerated radiotherapy. Radiother Oncol 2010;97(1): 86–91.

19. Logemann JA, Smith CH, Pauloski BR, et al. Effects of xerostomia on perception and performance of swallow function. Head Neck 2001;23(4):317–21.

20. Logemann JA, Pauloski BR, Rademaker AW, et al. Xerostomia: 12-month changes in saliva production and its relationship to perception and performance of swallow function, oral intake, and diet after chemoradiation. Head Neck 2003; 25(6):432–7.

21. Popovtzer A, Cao Y, Feng FY, et al. Anatomical changes in the pharyngeal constrictors after chemo-irradiation of head and neck cancer and their dose-effect relationships: MRI-based study. Radiother Oncol 2009;93(3):510–5.

22. Dornfeld K, Hopkins S, Simmons J, et al. Posttreatment FDG-PET uptake in the supraglottic and glottic larynx correlates with decreased quality of life after chemoradiotherapy. Int J Radiat Oncol Biol Phys 2008;71(2):386–92.

23. Feng FY, Kim HM, Lyden TH, et al. Intensity-modulated radiotherapy of head and neck cancer aiming to reduce dysphagia: early dose-effect relationships for the swallowing structures. Int J Radiat Oncol Biol Phys 2007;68(5):1289–98.

24. Levendag PC, Teguh DN, Voet P, et al. Dysphagia disorders in patients with cancer of the oropharynx are significantly affected by the radiation therapy dose to the superior and middle constrictor muscle: a dose-effect relationship. Radiother Oncol 2007;85(1):64–73.

25. Jensen K, Lambertsen K, Grau C. Late swallowing dysfunction and dysphagia after radiotherapy for pharynx cancer: frequency, intensity and correlation with dose and volume parameters. Radiother Oncol 2007;85(1):74–82.

26. Caglar HB, Tishler RB, Othus M, et al. Dose to larynx predicts for swallowing complications after intensity-modulated radiotherapy. Int J Radiat Oncol Biol Phys 2008;72(4):1110–8.

27. Rancati T, Schwarz M, Allen AM, et al. Radiation dose–volume effects in the larynx and pharynx. Int J Radiat Oncol Biol Phys 2010;76(Suppl 3):S64–9.

28. Ang KK, Trotti A, Brown BW, et al. Randomized trial addressing risk features and time factors of surgery plus radiotherapy in advanced head-and-neck cancer. Int J Radiat Oncol Biol Phys 2001;51(3):571–8.

29. Smith RV, Goldman SY, Beitler JJ, et al. Problems with altered radiotherapy dosing used in an organ-sparing protocol for advanced pharyngeal carcinoma. Arch Otolaryngol Head Neck Surg 2004;130(7):831–6.

30. Skladowski K, Maciejewski B, Golen M, et al. Randomized clinical trial on 7-day-continuous accelerated irradiation (CAIR) of head and neck cancer - report on 3-year tumour control and normal tissue toxicity. Radiother Oncol 2000;55(2):101–10.

31. Skladowski K, Maciejewski B, Golen M, et al. Continuous accelerated 7-days-a-week radiotherapy for head-and-neck cancer: long-term results of phase III clinical trial. Int J Radiat Oncol Biol Phys 2006;66(3):706–13.

32. Lauve A, Morris M, Schmidt-Ullrich R, et al. Simultaneous integrated boost intensity-modulated radiotherapy for locally advanced head-and-neck squamous cell carcinomas: II–clinical results. Int J Radiat Oncol Biol Phys 2004;60(2):374–87.

33. Koiwai K, Shikama N, Sasaki S, et al. Risk factors for severe Dysphagia after concurrent chemoradiotherapy for head and neck cancers. Jpn J Clin Oncol 2009;39(7):413–7.

34. Quon H, Leong T, Haselow R, et al. Phase III study of radiation therapy with or without cis-platinum in patients with unresectable squamous or undifferentiated carcinoma of the head and neck: an intergroup trial of the Eastern Cooperative Oncology Group (E2382). Int J Radiat Oncol Biol Phys 2011;81(3):719–25.

35. Bonner JA, Harari PM, Giralt J, et al. Radiotherapy plus cetuximab for squamous-cell carcinoma of the head and neck. N Engl J Med 2006;354(6):567–78.

36. Bonner JA, Harari PM, Giralt J, et al. Radiotherapy plus cetuximab for locoregionally advanced head and neck cancer: 5-year survival data from a phase 3 randomised trial, and relation between cetuximab-induced rash and survival. Lancet Oncol 2010;11(1):21–8.

37. Lango M, Ende K, Ahmad S, et al. Neck dissection following organ preservation protocols prolongs feeding tube dependence in patients with advanced head and neck cancer. J Clin Oncol (ASCO Meeting Abstracts) 2006;24(Suppl 18):5525.

38. Graner DE, Foote RL, Kasperbauer JL, et al. Swallow function in patients before and after intra-arterial chemoradiation. Laryngoscope 2003;113(3):573–9.

39. Chapuy CI, Annino DJ, Snavely A, et al. Swallowing function following postche-moradiotherapy neck dissection: review of findings and analysis of contributing factors. Otolaryngol Head Neck Surg 2011;145(3):428–34.

40. Carroll WR, Locher JL, Canon CL, et al. Pretreatment swallowing exercises improve swallow function after chemoradiation. Laryngoscope 2008;118(1): 39–43.

41. Ames JA, Karnell LH, Gupta AK, et al. Outcomes after the use of gastrostomy tubes in patients whose head and neck cancer was managed with radiation therapy. Head Neck 2011;33(5):638–44.

42. Dosoretz A, Dutta PR, Lin A, et al, editors. Long-term percutaneous gastrostomy tube dependence rates in patients treated with intensity-modulated radiotherapy for oropharyngeal cancer: the University of Pennsylvania Experience. ASTRO Head and Neck Symposium. Chandler (AZ); 2009.

43. Peponi E, Glanzmann C, Willi B, et al. Dysphagia in head and neck cancer patients following intensity modulated radiotherapy (IMRT). Radiat Oncol 2011; 6:1.

44. Moore EJ, Olsen KD, Kasperbauer JL. Transoral robotic surgery for oropharyn-geal squamous cell carcinoma: a prospective study of feasibility and functional outcomes. Laryngoscope 2009;119(11):2156–64.

45. Holsinger FC, McWhorter AJ, Menard M, et al. Transoral lateral oropharyngec-tomy for squamous cell carcinoma of the tonsillar region: I. Technique, complica-tions, and functional results. Arch Otolaryngol Head Neck Surg 2005;131(7): 583–91.

46. Bernier J, Domenge C, Ozsahin M, et al. Postoperative irradiation with or without concomitant chemotherapy for locally advanced head and neck cancer. N Engl J Med 2004;350(19):1945–52.

47. Cooper JS, Pajak TF, Forastiere AA, et al. Postoperative concurrent radiotherapy and chemotherapy for high-risk squamous-cell carcinoma of the head and neck. N Engl J Med 2004;350(19):1937–44.

48. Weinstein GS, Quon H, O'Malley BW Jr, et al. Selective neck dissection and de-intensified postoperative radiation and chemotherapy for oropharyngeal cancer: a subset analysis of the University of Pennsylvania TORS trial. Laryngoscope 2010;120(9):1749–55.

49. O'Sullivan B, Warde P, Grice B, et al. The benefits and pitfalls of ipsilateral radio-therapy in carcinoma of the tonsillar region. Int J Radiat Oncol Biol Phys 2001; 51(2):332–43.

Rehabilitation Needs of Patients with Oropharyngeal Cancer

Donna C. Tippett, MPH, MA, CCC-SLP[a,b],
Kimberly T. Webster, MA, MS, CCC-SLP[a,*]

KEYWORDS

- Dysphagia • Xerostomia • HPV-related oropharyngeal cancer • Swallowing
- Functional outcomes • Quality of life

KEY POINTS

- There are multiple and varied functional deficits related to swallowing resulting from oropharyngeal cancer and organ preservation treatment approaches. These deficits encompass diminished quality of life, weight loss, xerostomia, and need for gastrostomy tube.
- Findings from instrumental videofluoroscopic swallow studies of individuals with head and neck cancer include deficits in oral, pharyngeal, and esophageal phases of swallowing. These deficits include reduced base-of-tongue retraction, reduced pharyngeal constriction, reduced laryngeal elevation, laryngeal penetration or aspiration, pharyngeal retention of boluses, and reduced cricopharyngeal opening.
- Interventional strategies to help individuals with oropharyngeal cancer maximize functional outcomes related to swallowing, including pretreatment education regarding anticipated effects on speech or voice and swallowing. These include, but are not limited to, information about xerostomia, oral hygiene, trismus and prophylactic swallowing, and jaw range-of-motion exercises.
- Initial examination of differences between individuals with human papillomavirus (HPV)-related and HPV-nonrelated oropharyngeal cancer reveals no statistically significant differences; however, patients with HPV-related cancer had fewer swallowing deficits and earlier removal of feeding tubes.
- Given the prevalence of dysphagia in this population, the authors advocate for pretreatment intervention by speech-language pathologists for individuals diagnosed with head and neck cancer.

We declare that we have no conflicts of interest in the authorship or publication of this contribution.
a Department of Otolaryngology-Head and Neck Surgery, Johns Hopkins University School of Medicine, Baltimore, MD, USA; b Department of Physical Medicine and Rehabilitation, Johns Hopkins University School of Medicine, Baltimore, MD, USA
* Corresponding author. Department of Otolaryngology-Head and Neck Surgery, 601 North Caroline Street, JHOC 6th Floor, Baltimore, MD 21287-0910.
E-mail address: kwebste1@jhmi.edu

Otolaryngol Clin N Am 45 (2012) 863–878
doi:10.1016/j.otc.2012.05.005
0030-6665/12/$ – see front matter © 2012 Elsevier Inc. All rights reserved.

oto.theclinics.com

Abbreviations: Rehabilitation for Oropharyngeal Cancer Patients	
DTS	Dynasplint® Trismus System
MID	Maximal interincisal distance
PEG	Percutaneous endoscopic gastrostomy
RADPLAT	Radiation plus cisplatin
VFSS	Videofluoroscopic swallowing studies

INTRODUCTION

The favorable oncologic outcomes of organ preservation therapy for individuals with head and neck cancer are well-established.[1–6] Increasingly, individuals with head and neck cancer are being treated with organ preservation approaches rather than surgery. Nonsurgical approaches include:

- Radiation therapy alone
- Neoadjuvant chemotherapy with radiation
- Induction chemotherapy
- Concurrent chemoradiation treatment.

Preservation of structure afforded by these management options, unfortunately, does not correlate with preservation of function. Posttreatment dysphagia, dysphonia, and related complications are described in multiple sources.[7–13] Increased radiation dose to a larger volume of the pharyngeal constrictors is associated with more severe dysphagia, resulting in diminished quality of life after treatment.[14–16] In this article, evaluation and treatment of dysphagia in individuals receiving chemoradiation and radiation to treat their head and neck cancer at Johns Hopkins Hospital are presented. Pretreatment and posttreatment speech-language pathology evaluation is described, including specific swallowing deficits and interventions to address these deficits. Evidence regarding the role of oral motor exercises, management of trismus, treatment of xerostomia, and the influence of oral hygiene are reviewed. In addition, clinical outcomes of patients whose tumors are human papillomavirus (HPV)-related and HPV-nonrelated are compared.

VIDEOFLUOROSCOPIC FINDINGS IN INDIVIDUALS TREATED WITH CHEMORADIATION AND/OR RADIATION THERAPY

Dysphagia in patients treated with chemoradiation and radiation is characterized by a multiplicity of deficits. Several investigators have reported objective findings from videofluoroscopic swallowing studies (VFSS). Similar findings have been documented by the investigators. For example, Lazarus and colleagues[17] conducted VFSS in nine patients with head and neck cancer who were treated with radiation therapy and adjuvant chemotherapy. They reported aspiration, reduced posterior tongue base retraction, reduced laryngeal elevation, and need for multiple swallows to clear pharyngeal residue. Carrara-de Angelis and colleagues[18] conducted VFSS to assess 14 patients who were treated with concomitant paclitaxel, cisplatin, and radiotherapy for advanced squamous cell carcinoma of the larynx or hypopharynx. Findings included

- Reduced bolus formation (n = 13)
- Reduced bolus propulsion (n = 12)

- Oral stasis (n = 13)
- Pharyngeal stasis (n = 12)
- Reduced laryngeal elevation (n = 5).

Patients were rated using the Penetration-Aspiration Scale[19]:

- There was no penetration or aspiration in three patients
- Penetration occurred in six patients
- Aspiration occurred in five patients.

Most patients received swallowing therapy after the VFSS. At follow-up (mean 20 months, range 10–32 months)

- 7 of the 14 patients had normal swallowing
- 1 patient was still using a gastrostomy feeding tube.

Lazarus[20] assessed lingual strength and conducted VFSS in 12 patients who were treated with radiotherapy:

- All subjects demonstrated tongue strength impairment and had reduced base-of-tongue retraction on the video studies.

Pretreatment and posttreatment swallowing function has been described in multiple sources:

- Eisbruch and colleagues[21] conducted VFSS of patients with locally advanced head and neck cancer before and after chemoradiation therapy. Swallowing function was not normal before treatment, which was most likely due to location of the tumors in the upper digestive tract. Furthermore, multiple swallowing decompensations were identified after treatment in the absence of bulky tumor; six patients developed pneumonia that was attributed to aspiration.
- Pauloski and colleagues[22] performed VFSS on 352 patients with head and neck cancer who were to receive either primary surgery or primary radiation therapy with or without concurrent chemotherapy. Similar to Eisbruch and colleagues,[21] their findings showed that the presence of a tumor in the upper aerodigestive track can disrupt normal swallowing. Patients with oral cavity and pharyngeal lesions tended to have poorer swallow function than those with laryngeal lesions. Patients with laryngeal tumors had significantly shorter oral transit times, less oral residue, shorter pharyngeal transit times, and longer cricopharyngeal opening than did those with either oral or pharyngeal lesions.
- Graner and colleagues[23] evaluated swallowing in 11 patients with advanced head and neck cancer before and after completion of intraarterial chemoradiation and planned neck dissection. On the pretreatment VFSS, swallow function was impaired in 9 of 11 patients, with aspiration seen in 3 patients. Following treatment, aspiration was observed in 7 patients. Tongue base retraction, reduced laryngeal elevation, and increased laryngeal vestibule penetration of thick liquid were all statistically significantly worse after treatment. After treatment, soft diets were required and ability to eat in public was restricted.
- Kotz and colleagues[24] also conducted before and after chemoradiation and chemoradiation VFSS in patients with advanced-stage head and neck cancer. On the posttreatment studies, all patients had reduced contact between base of tongue and posterior pharyngeal wall. Most patients also had reduced laryngeal elevation and compromised laryngeal vestibule closure.

- Logemann and colleagues[10] evaluated 53 patients with advanced head and neck cancer before and 3 months after completing chemoradiation treatment. Findings were reported by site of the primary cancer. Before treatment, 28% of the patients with laryngeal cancer had gastrostomy tubes and 14% were aspirating. Three months after treatment, the laryngeal cancer group had the highest frequency of reduced base-of-tongue retraction, reduced anterior-posterior tongue movement, delayed pharyngeal swallow, reduced laryngeal elevation, and reduced cricopharyngeal opening compared with the nasopharyngeal, oropharyngeal, hypopharyngeal, and unknown primary cancer groups. Furthermore, half of these patients continued to use their gastrostomy feeding tubes posttreatment and 7% continued to aspirate.

FUNCTIONAL OUTCOMES IN INDIVIDUALS TREATED WITH CHEMORADIATION AND/OR RADIATION THERAPY

Murry and colleagues[25] evaluated quality of life and swallowing in 58 patients who were treated with chemoradiation:

- Swallowing status was decreased during and immediately after treatment compared with pretreatment levels.
- At the 6-month evaluation, quality of life returned to pretreatment levels, but swallowing status remained slightly below baseline.

Newman and colleagues[26] described eating changes and weight loss in 47 individuals with advanced head and neck cancer treated with an intraarterial-administered chemoradiation protocol (radiation plus cisplatin [RADPLAT]):

- Subjects lost 10% of their pretreatment weight and had deterioration in eating ability over the course of treatment.
- At 18 months posttreatment, six patients still required percutaneous endoscopic gastrostomy (PEG) tubes and 34 reported normal or near-normal eating ability.
- In a follow up study, intraarterial (RADPLAT) and intravenous-administered chemoradiation patients did not differ significantly on most swallow outcome measures at 1 month posttreatment, although there was significantly less aspiration on small bolus volumes in the RADPLAT group.[27]

Gillespie and colleagues[7] surveyed 22 patients with head and neck cancer who were treated with surgery followed by postoperative radiation and 18 treated with chemoradiation regarding quality of life:

- Patients who received chemoradiation for oropharyngeal primaries demonstrated significantly better scores on the emotional and functional scales on the MD Anderson Dysphagia Inventory[28] than did patients who underwent surgery followed by radiation therapy.
- In contrast, there were no significant differences in subscale score for the surgery or radiation and chemoradiation groups for laryngeal or hypopharyngeal cancer sites.

Mowery and colleagues[29] assessed quality of life in 17 patients with oropharyngeal cancer and 14 patients with laryngeal cancer status after chemoradiation. Mean time from completion of chemoradiation to assessment was 11 months:

- Patients with oropharyngeal cancer reported diminished saliva significantly more often than the patients with laryngeal cancer.

- Both groups reported difficulty with swallowing, chewing, and taste. Swallowing difficulties were attributed to tissue edema, friability, and fibrosis.
- Nine of the patients with 14 laryngeal cancer and 6 of the 17 patients with oropharyngeal cancer rated quality of life as "good" or better.

Goguen and colleagues[9] periodically assessed the swallowing status of 54 patients with head and neck cancer who received chemoradiation:

- All patients developed dysphagia and had weight loss.
- At 1 year follow-up, 80% were taking a soft diet and 81% had their gastrostomy feeding tube removed.
- At 2 years posttreatment, 97% were taking a soft diet and 90% had their gastrostomy feeding tube removed, highlighting the need for long term follow-up.

IATROGENIC COMPLICATIONS

Several side-effects associated with radiotherapy and chemotherapy have implications for swallowing. A primary complication of chemotherapy is mucositis,[30] which can persist for weeks following completion of treatment, causing oral and pharyngeal tenderness and pain as well as sensitivity to temperature and spicy or acidic foods. Complications associated with radiotherapy can be acute or late onset and include[31,32]

- Mucositis
- Candidiasis
- Dysgeusia
- Dental caries
- Osteoradionecrosis
- Soft tissue necrosis
- Xerostomia.

Intensity-modulated radiation therapy provides a highly conformal dose distribution around tumor targets and potentially spares normal mucosa and salivary glands.[33] Medications may also be used either to protect salivary glands or to improve salivary flow.[34,35] Dentifrices can be used to ameliorate dry mouth. Patients should be counseled to maintain some degree of oral intake during and after treatment to avoid stricture formation.[36]

Trismus or Mandibular Hypomobility

Trismus or mandibular hypomobility[37] occurs in 5% to 38% of patients with head and neck cancer, with wide variation attributed to the lack of uniform criteria for diagnosis, visual assessment, and retrospective assessment.[38] Normal maximal incisal opening is 45 ± 7 mm.[39] Dijkstra and colleagues,[38] and Buchbinder and colleagues.[40] defined less than 30 to 35 mm as the functional cut off for trismus in oncology patients. Trismus has implications for oral hygiene, biting, chewing, speaking, laughing, yawning, airway management, and oral cancer surveillance.

Trismus can be treated with range of movement exercises, stacked tongue blades, and specialized medical devices:

- Botulinum toxin injections into the masseter muscles of postradiation patients have shown an improvement in pain symptoms associated with trismus, but no improvement in oral aperture.[41]
- The Therabite (Atos Medical Inc, WI, USA) is a hand-operated device that uses passive motion to address jaw hypomobility and dysfunction. Buchbinder and

colleagues[40] reported that individuals who were treated using the Therabite had significant increase in maximal incisal opening compared with those who were treated with range of movement exercises and stacked tongue blades. Cohen and colleagues[42] found significant increases in maximal incisal opening in patients' status after surgery for oropharyngeal squamous cell cancer who used the Therabite.

- The Dynasplint Trismus System (DTS) (Dynasplint systems Inc, MD, USA) is a device that uses low-load prolonged-duration stretch and has been shown to reduce contracture and improve range of motion in muscles of mastication in patients with trismus. Patients with trismus related to radiation therapy, dental treatment, oral surgery, and stroke used the device for 20 to 30 minutes, 3 times per day, and showed increased maximal interincisal distance (MID) with a mean change for all groups of 12.8 mm.[43] Similarly, Stubblefield and colleagues[41] demonstrated that the DTS used 30 minutes, 3 times per day, was effective in increasing MID in a group of 20 patients with trismus after head and neck cancer combined modality treatment. Compliant patients increased MID from 16 to 27 mm ($P<.001$).

It is well-known that dysphagia is a necessary but not sufficient condition to cause aspiration pneumonia. Other risk factors must be present and have been shown to be significant predictors of aspiration pneumonia in elderly patients with dysphagia. Some of these include[44]

- Dependency for oral care
- Number of decayed teeth
- Smoking.

More specific dental and oral risk factors for aspiration pneumonia have been identified in a study of an elderly veteran population by Terpenning and colleagues.[45] These include:

- Number of decayed teeth
- Number of functional dental units
- Periodontal disease
- Presence of organisms for decay, specifically, *Streptococcus sabrinus* and *Staphylococcus aureus* in saliva, and *Porphyromonas gingivalis* in dental plaque.

Counseling on oral hygiene is an essential component of dysphagia education for all dysphagia patients but especially for those undergoing organ preservation treatment of head and neck cancer because oral mucositis and xerostomia have been found to occur in nearly 100% of these patients.[35,46]

SPEECH-LANGUAGE PATHOLOGY TREATMENT PROTOCOL

At Johns Hopkins Hospital, individuals undergoing organ preservation approaches are treated by a multidisciplinary team. The treatment protocol begins at Tumor Board Conferences. Individuals with head and neck cancer are presented at weekly Tumor Board Conferences, which are multidisciplinary treatment planning meetings attended by head and neck surgeons, medical oncologists, radiation oncologists, oral pathologists, oncology and otolaryngology nurses, speech-language pathologists, dental prosthodontists, and nuclear medicine radiologists.

Pretreatment Evaluation and Education

Speech-language pathologists meet with patients before initiation of radiation or chemoradiation and evaluate patients posttreatment. Evidence supports the importance of pretreatment education as critical to long-term rehabilitation outcomes.[47] Patients are also seen approximately 4 weeks into radiation therapy to reevaluate and review or initiate other exercises as necessary. They may be seen more frequently as needed.

During the pretreatment visit, expected changes that may affect speech, voice, or swallowing are reviewed. Routine and professional dental care and consultations with dentists, oral pathologists, and prosthodontists are recommended, as appropriate, for medical and pharmaceutical management of radiation and chemoradiation side effects. Other research-proven treatment methods, such as acupuncture, may also be discussed and appropriate referrals made with medical consent. Pretreatment swallowing exercises, shown to be associated with improved quality of life,[48,49] are initiated. Counseling about xerostomia and oral hygiene is a vital educational component. Speech-language pathologists offer strategies and treatments to minimize the impact of trismus, which can result in significant morbidity. Baseline oral aperture is measured.

Patients are followed during their treatment as needed.

Posttreatment Evaluation

Posttreatment VFSS are conducted and swallowing treatment regimen may be modified based on the VFSS results. Oral motor exercises, derived from speech and voice literature, have been a mainstay of dysphagia treatment to increase strength, endurance, and power. Ideally, oral motor exercises are selected based on an evidence-based approach, incorporating research evidence, clinical expertise, and patient values.[50] Rigorous, client-specific research is limited at this point in speech-language pathology; however, clinicians can look to cohort and case series to play a complimentary role in the treatment planning process along with their clinical expertise and knowledge of anatomy and physiology. Oral motor exercises can be selected based on the exercise physiology principles of goal selection, specificity of training, and overload or progression,[51] as well as on deficits expected based on disease site.[10]

Posttreatment evaluation and VFSS in particular may also reveal the need for additional medical or surgical interventions. Gastroenterologists and laryngologists are part of the dysphagia team at Johns Hopkins Hospital. There is sometimes a role for endoscopy and cricopharyngeal-esophageal dilatation if webs, rings, and strictures are identified during videofluoroscopy. Additionally, vocal fold injection or augmentation, as well as medialization, may improve vocal fold closure, contributing to better airway protection for swallowing purposes, as well as improved voice (**Table 1**).[52]

JOHNS HOPKINS' EXPERIENCE

The authors conducted a retrospective study of patients with oropharyngeal cancer treated with chemoradiation, comparing swallowing results in HPV-related and HPV-nonrelated disease.

Methods

Before initiation of the study, the data collection, review, and analysis were approved by the Johns Hopkins Medicine Institutional Review Board. Candidates for inclusion were individuals with head and neck cancer undergoing radiation or chemoradiation. These were consecutive referrals.

- There were 53 patients; 42 were men.
- Race was: 46 white, 4 African American, 1 Asian, 1 Hispanic, and 1 Middle Eastern.

Table 1
Johns Hopkins hospital speech-language pathology approach to head and neck cancer treatment

Information Provided	Pretreatment	4th Wk of Radiation	2 Wk Postradiation	2 Mo Postradiation	6 Mo Postradiation
Review of normal voice and swallowing	√	—	—	—	—
General information about chemoradiation side effects	√	—	—	—	—
Importance of oral hygiene, dental care, and relation to mucositis and xerostomia	√	√	√	√	√
Inquiry about xerostomia and suggestions to alleviate symptoms	√	√	√	√	√
Trismus explanation, measurement of oral aperture	√	√	√	√	√
Jaw range-of-motion exercises for prevention or reduction of trismus	√	√	prn	prn	prn
Therapy with an antitrismus device	—	—	prn	prn	—
Clinical swallow evaluation	√	prn	√	prn	prn
Instrumental swallow evaluation (FEES or VFSS)	prn	—	√	prn	prn
Additional oral motor exercises	prn	prn	prn	prn	prn
Dysphagia exercises	√	√	prn	prn	prn
Referrals for medical-surgical dysphagia or voice intervention	—	—	prn	prn	prn

Abbreviations: FEES, fiberoptic endoscopic evaluation of swallowing; prn, pro re nata.

- Mean age was 57.3 years (range 22–81 years).
- Diagnoses were: 50 oropharyngeal squamous cell carcinoma, 2 nasopharyngeal carcinoma, and 1 unknown primary.
- Thirty-eight patients were HPV-positive, 11 were HPV-negative, and 4 were unknown or not tested.

Table 2
Pretreatment status denying dysphagia

	All	HPV-positive	HPV-negative	HPV-unknown
Denied dysphagia	30:53	24:38	4:11	2:4
	57%	63%	36%	50%

All patients were evaluated by a speech-language pathologist before chemoradiation. Patients were followed during their treatment as needed. VFSS were conducted with a radiologist, radiology technologist, and speech-language pathologist. Boluses included thin liquid barium (Barosperse Barium Sulfate), thick liquid (E-Z-HD Barium Sulfate), applesauce with barium paste (Intropaste Barium Sulfate Paste), and graham cracker with barium paste. Bolus types and amounts (graded and ungraded) were given based on clinical status and radiographic information. Studies were reviewed by the radiologist and speech-language pathologist. Separate reports were generated by the radiologist and speech-language pathologist.

Data were collected from the speech-language pathologist evaluation reports and the radiology reports for the following videofluoroscopic observations:

1. Velopharyngeal apposition
2. Base-of-tongue retraction
3. Epiglottic tilt
4. Hyoid elevation
5. Airway protection
6. Reflexive cough
7. Pharyngeal constriction
8. Pharyngeal clearance
9. Cricopharyngeal function
10. Esophageal function.

Results

All subjects
At pretreatment, 30 of 53 (57%) patients denied dysphagia (**Table 2**). Of those who reported signs or symptoms of dysphagia, the most frequent pretreatment complaints were (**Table 3**):

- Cough or choke 9 of 53 (17%)
- Odynophagia 10 of 53 (19%)
- Diet change 11 of 53 (21%).

Infrequent pretreatment complaints were (**Table 4**):

Table 3
Most frequent pretreatment dysphagia complaints

Most Frequent Complaints	All	HPV-positive	HPV-negative	HPV-unknown
Cough or choke	9:53	7:38	2:11	0
	17%	18%	18%	
Odynophagia	10:53	5:38	3:11	2:4
	19%	13%	27%	50%
Diet change	11:53	6:38	5:11	0
	21%	16%	45%	

Table 4
Infrequent pretreatment dysphagia complaints

Infrequent Complaints	All	HPV-positive	HPV-negative	HPV-unknown
Nasal regurgitation	1:53	1:38	0	0
	2%	3%		
Reduced oral control	2:53	1:38	1:11	0
	4%	3%	9%	
Trismus	5:53	4:38	1:11	0
	9%	11%	9%	
Weight loss	7:53	4:38	2:11	1:4
	13%	11%	18%	25%

- Nasal regurgitation 1 of 53 (2%)
- Reduced oral control 2 of 53 (4%)
- Trismus 5 of 53 (9%)
- Weight loss 7 of 53 (13%).

Specific impairments on the videofluoroscopic swallowing studies were as follows (**Table 5**):

- Epiglottic tilt 39 of 53 (74%)
- Pharyngeal constriction 39 of 53 (74%)
- Pharyngeal clearance 39 of 53 (74%)
- Airway protection 31 of 53 (58%)
- Hyoid elevation 24 of 53 (45%)
- Cricopharyngeal function 22 of 53 (42%)
- Two patients (both HPV-positive) presented with no deficits on VFSS
- Three patients (two HPV-positive) had esophageal strictures.

All patients were rated on the Penetration-Aspiration Scale.[19] There was a bimodal distribution of ratings (**Fig 1**). The relationship between presence of a PEG at 3 months and Penetration-Aspiration Scale score was analyzed with the following

Table 5
Posttreatment VFSS results: most frequent findings by site

Frequency of Impairment by Site	All	HPV-positive	HPV-negative	HPV-unknown
Epiglottic tilt	39:53	26:38	9:11	4:4
	74%	68%	82%	100%
Pharyngeal constriction	39:53	25:38	10:11	4:4
	74%	66%	91%	100%
Pharyngeal clearance	39:53	26:38	9:11	4:4
	74%	68%	82%	100%
Airway protection	31:53	21:38	6:11	4:4
	58%	55%	55%	100%
Hyoid elevation	24:53	18:38	4:11	2:4
	45%	47%	36%	50%
Cricopharyngeal function	22:53	15:38	6:11	1:4
	42%	39%	55%	25%

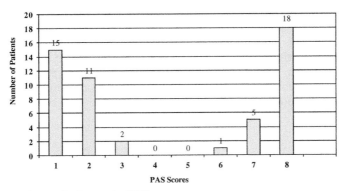

Fig. 1. Penetration-aspiration scale (PAS) scores.

results: sensitivity = 72%, specificity = 61%, positive predictive value = 70%, negative predictive value = 64%, and odds ratio = 4.1.

After treatment (**Table 6**):

- Xerostomia was present at greater than 6 months posttreatment in 51 of 53 (96%)
- Trismus was present in 13 of 53(25%)
- The PEG tube was removed by 3-months posttreatment in 23 of 53 (43%) and by 6-months posttreatment in 32 of 51 (60%).

HPV-positive versus HPV-negative patients

Results were analyzed comparing HPV-positive versus HPV-negative patients:

- More HPV-positive patients denied dysphagia symptoms before treatment than HPV-negative patients (63% HPV-positive vs 36% HPV-negative) (see **Table 2**).
- Higher percentages of HPV-negative patients reported odynophagia and need for diet change, the latter reaching statistical significance at $P = .05$ ($X^2 = 4.312$, $df = 1$, $3.841 < P < 6.635$) (see **Table 3**).
- Percentages were similar for both groups for infrequent complaints of nasal regurgitation, reduced oral control, trismus, and weight loss (see **Table 4**).
- Regarding differences in posttreatment VFSS results, there were higher percentages of impairments (by site) in the HPV-negative group for four out of the six most frequent dysphagia problems (epiglottic tilt, pharyngeal constriction,

Table 6
Posttreatment status results for xerostomia, trismus, and PEG removal

	All	HPV-positive	HPV-negative	HPV-unknown
Xerostomia 6–12 mo	51:53 96%	36:38 95%	11:11 100%	4:4 100%
Trismus	13:53 25%	8:38 21%	3:11 27%	2:4 59%
PEG removed 3 mo	23:53 43%	18:38 47%	4:11 36%	1:4 25%
PEG removed 6 mo	32:53% 60%	25:38 66%	6:11 55%	1:4 25%

pharyngeal clearance, and cricopharyngeal function) (see **Table 5**). These differences were not statistically significant.

- After treatment, xerostomia and trismus were similarly prevalent in patients regardless of HPV status, although a higher percentage of the HPV-unknown status patients had posttreatment trismus. A higher, though statistically insignificant, number of HPV-positive patients had feeding tubes removed by 3 and 6 months posttreatment (see **Table 6**).

SUMMARY

Based on review of the literature and the outcomes of the 53 Johns Hopkins patients, several recommendations can be made regarding treatment of dysphagia and related impairments for patients with oropharyngeal cancer:

- Approximately half of the John Hopkins patients reported pretreatment dysphagia. Complaints centered on coughing or choking, odynophagia, and need for diet change. These findings reinforce the need to query patients about pretreatment swallowing status and to use a multidisciplinary approach.
- One-fourth of the John Hopkins patients reported a need to modify their diet at baseline, highlighting the need for dietary or nutrition input early in the diagnosis-treatment paradigm. Absence of pretreatment dysphagia is not predictive of posttreatment dysphagia, underscoring the need for early intervention to address anticipated swallowing-related difficulties.
- Pretreatment intervention, including thorough education, baseline assessment of swallowing, and nutrition and initiation of prophylactic swallowing and oral motor exercises seems to benefit this patient population. Primary topics addressed in the pretreatment evaluation at Johns Hopkins Hospital by the speech pathology division in Otolaryngology-Head and Neck Surgery include xerostomia, oral hygiene, trismus, dysphagia (prevention or intervention), temporary taste and appetite changes, and importance of adequate nutrition and hydration. Attention is given to distinguishing between temporary taste and appetite changes versus true dysphagia:
- Pharyngeal impairments were common in the John Hopkins patients on posttreatment VFSS. These findings were consistent with reports by other investigators.[10,17–24] The John Hopkins protocol includes prophylactic swallowing exercises that address pharyngeal function.[48,49] Multiplicity of posttreatment swallowing problems did not preclude oral intake during treatment. Almost half had the PEG tube removed by 3 months. Presence of a PEG tube is not an indicator of swallowing or oral intake status, although there was an association between aspiration and PEG at 3 months.
- One-fourth had trismus posttreatment, and nearly everyone had xerostomia. These swallowing-related issues are known to impact quality of life and clearly need to be addressed during pretreatment counseling and treated as indicated by appropriate team members during and after oncologic interventions.
- Clinically indicative data favored functional swallowing outcomes of HPV-positive patients, although only need for diet change pretreatment reached statistical significance. Lack of statistically significant findings may be a reflection of small sample size, or may not be expected; dysphagia in these patients is secondary to chemoradiation and may not be influenced by the causes of tumor.

Further exploration of potential differences between HPV-positive and HPV-negative populations is needed as the field explores de-escalation protocols for HPV-related head and neck cancers aimed to improve quality of life.

FUTURE DIRECTIONS

Future directions for research include determining clinical correlates of dysphagia severity, investigating compliance with treatment recommendations, exploring barriers to compliance, and examining relationship of oral intake status and dysphagia. Future studies with larger subject samples should seek to examine a correlation and exact relationship between pretreatment exercises and posttreatment function. At this time, however, this protocol seems promising in helping individuals with head and neck cancer undergoing chemoradiation achieve maximum function and quality of life. Advocacy of pretreatment evaluation and initiation of prophylactic oral and pharyngeal exercises, meeting with patients as necessary during chemoradiation treatments, and follow-up after treatment with instrumental dysphagia evaluations and appropriate intervention continues to be warranted.

REFERENCES

1. Department of Veterans Affairs Laryngeal Cancer Study Group. Induction chemotherapy plus radiation compared with surgery plus radiation in patients with advanced laryngeal cancer: the Department of Veterans Affairs Laryngeal Cancer Study Group. N Engl J Med 1991;324(24):1685–90.
2. Forastiere AA, Goepfert H, Maor M, et al. Concurrent chemotherapy and radiotherapy for organ preservation in advanced laryngeal cancer. N Engl J Med 2003;349(22):2091–8.
3. Bourhis J, Overgaard J, Audry H, et al. Hyperfractionated or accelerated radiotherapy in head and neck cancer: a meta-analysis. Lancet 2006;368(9538):843–54.
4. Garden AS, Harris J, Trotti A, et al. Long-term results of concomitant boost radiation plus concurrent cisplatin for advanced head and neck carcinomas: a phase II trial of the radiation therapy oncology group (RTOG 99-14). Int J Radiat Oncol Biol Phys 2008;71(5):1351–5.
5. Nuyts S, Dirix P, Clement PM, et al. Impact of adding concomitant chemotherapy to hyperfractionated accelerated radiotherapy for advanced head and neck squamous cell carcinoma. Int J Radiat Oncol Biol Phys 2009;73(4):1088–95.
6. Pignon JP, le Maitre A, Maillard E, et al. Meta-analysis of chemotherapy in head and neck cancer (MACH-NC): an update on 93 randomised trials and 17,346 patients. Radiother Oncol 2009;92(1):4–14.
7. Gillespie MB, Brodsky MB, Day TA, et al. Swallowing-related quality of life after head and neck cancer treatment. Laryngoscope 2004;114(8):1362–7.
8. Dworkin JP, Hill SL, Stachler RJ, et al. Swallowing function outcomes following nonsurgical therapy for advanced-stage laryngeal carcinoma. Dysphagia 2006; 21(1):66–74.
9. Goguen LA, Posner MR, Norris CM, et al. Dysphagia after sequential chemoradiation therapy for advanced head and neck cancer. Otolaryngol Head Neck Surg 2006;134(6):916–22.
10. Logemann JA, Rademaker AW, Pauloski BR, et al. Site of disease and treatment protocol as correlates of swallowing function in patients with head and neck cancer treated with chemoradiation. Head Neck 2006;28(1):64–73.
11. Nguyen NP, Frank C, Moltz CC, et al. Aspiration rate following chemoradiation for head and neck cancer: an underreported occurrence. Radiother Oncol 2006; 80(3):302–6.
12. Logemann JA, Pauloski BR, Rademaker AW, et al. Swallowing disorders in the first year after definitive radiation and chemoradiation. Head Neck 2008;30(2): 148–58.

13. Caudell JJ, Schaner PE, Meredith RF, et al. Factors associated with long-term dysphagia after definitive radiotherapy for locally advanced head and neck cancer. Int J Radiat Oncol Biol Phys 2009;73(2):410–5.

14. Feng FY, Kim HM, Lyden TH, et al. Intensity-modulated radiotherapy of head and neck cancer aiming to reduce dysphagia: early-dose effect relationship for the swallowing structures. Int J Radiat Oncol Biol Phys 2007;68(5):1289–98.

15. Caglar HB, Tishler RB, Othus M, et al. Dose to larynx predicts for swallowing complications after intensity-modulated radiotherapy. Int J Radiat Oncol Biol Phys 2008;72(4):1110–8.

16. Caudell JJ, Schaner PE, Desmond RA, et al. Dosimetric factors associated with long-term dysphagia after radiotherapy for squamous cell carcinoma of the head and neck. Int J Radiat Oncol Biol Phys 2010;76(2):403–9.

17. Lazarus C, Logemann J, Pauloski B, et al. Swallowing disorders in head and neck cancer patients treated with radiotherapy and adjuvant chemotherapy. Laryngoscope 1996;106(9 Pt 1):1157–66.

18. Carrara-de Angelis E, Feher O, Barros AP, et al. Voice and swallowing in patients enrolled in a larynx preservation trial. Arch Otolaryngol Head Neck Surg 2003; 129(7):733–8.

19. Rosenbek JC, Robbins J, Roecker EB, et al. A penetration-aspiration scale. Dysphagia 1996;11(2):93–8.

20. Lazarus C. Tongue strength and exercise in healthy individuals and head and neck cancer patients. Semin Speech Lang 2006;27(4):260–7.

21. Eisbruch A, Lyden T, Bradford CR, et al. Objective assessment of swallowing dysfunction and aspiration after radiation concurrent with chemotherapy for head-and-neck cancer. Int J Radiat Oncol Biol Phys 2002;53(1):23–8.

22. Pauloski BR, Rademaker AW, Logemann JA, et al. Pretreatment swallowing function in patients with head and neck cancer. Head Neck 2000;22(5): 474–82.

23. Graner DE, Foote RL, Kasperbauer JL, et al. Swallow function in patients before and after intra-arterial chemoradiation. Laryngoscope 2003;113(3):573–9.

24. Kotz T, Costello R, Li Y, et al. Swallowing dysfunction after chemoradiation for advanced squamous cell carcinoma of the head and neck. Head Neck 2004; 26(4):365–72.

25. Murry T, Madasu R, Martin A, et al. Acute and chronic changes in swallowing and quality of life following intraarterial chemoradiation for organ preservation in patients with advanced head and neck cancer. Head Neck 1998;20:31–7.

26. Newman LA, Vieira F, Schwierzer V, et al. Eating and weight changes following chemoradiation therapy for advanced head and neck cancer. Arch Otolaryngol Head Neck Surg 1998;124(5):589–92.

27. Newman LA, Robbins T, Logemann JA, et al. Swallowing and speech ability after treatment for head and neck cancer with targeted intraarterial versus intravenous chemoradiation. Head Neck 2002;24(1):68–77.

28. Chen AY, Frankowski R, Bishop-Leone J, et al. The development and validation of a dysphagia-specific quality-of-life questionnaire for patient with head and neck cancer. Arch Otolaryngol Head Neck Surg 2001;127(7):870–6.

29. Mowery SE, LoTempio MM, Sadeghi A, et al. Quality of life outcomes in laryngeal and oropharyngeal cancer patients after chemoradiation. Otolaryngol Head Neck Surg 2006;135(4):565–70.

30. Jacobs C, Goffinet D, Goffinet L, et al. Chemotherapy as a substitute for surgery in the treatment of advanced resectable head and neck cancer. Cancer 1987; 60(6):1178–83.

31. Jbam BC, da Silva Freire AR. Oral complications of radiotherapy in the head and neck. Rev Bras Otorrinolaringol 2006;72(5):704–8.
32. Dirix P, Nuyts S. Evidence-based organ-sparing radiotherapy in head and neck cancer. Lancet Oncol 2010;11(1):85–91.
33. Eisbruch A, Schwartz M, Rasch C, et al. Dysphagia and aspiration after chemo-radiotherapy for head-and-neck cancer: which anatomic structures are affected and can they be spared by IMRT? Int J Radiat Oncol Biol Phys 2004;60(5): 1425–39.
34. Brizel DM, Wasserman TH, Henke M, et al. Phase III randomized trial of amifostine as a radioprotector in head and neck cancer. J Clin Oncol 2000;18(19): 3339–45.
35. Johnstone PA, Peng YP, May BC, et al. Acupuncture for pilocarpine resistant xerostomia following radiotherapy for head and neck malignancies. Int J Radiat Oncol Biol Phys 2001;50(2):353–7.
36. Kotz T, Abraham S, Beitler JJ, et al. Pharyngeal transport dysfunction consequent to an organ-sparing protocol. Arch Otolaryngol Head Neck Surg 1999;125(4):410–3.
37. O'Leary MR. Trismus: modern pathophysiological correlates. Am J Emerg Med 1990;8(3):220–7.
38. Dijkstra PU, Huisman PM, Roodenburg JL. Criteria for trismus in head and neck oncology. Int J Oral Maxillofac Surg 2006;35(4):337–42.
39. Steelman R, Sokol J. Quantification of trismus following irradiation of the temporomandibular joint. Mo Dent J 1986;66(6):21–3.
40. Buchbinder D, Currivan RB, Kaplan AJ, et al. Mobilization regimens for the prevention of jaw hypomobility in the radiated patient: a comparison of three techniques. J Oral Maxillofac Surg 1993;51(8):863–7.
41. Stubblefield MD, Manfield L, Riedel ER. A preliminary report on the efficacy of a dynamic jaw opening device (dynasplint trismus system) as part of the multimodal treatment of trismus in patients with head and neck cancer. Arch Phys Med Rehabil 2010;91(8):1278–82.
42. Cohen EG, Deschler DG, Walsh K, et al. Early use of a mechanical stretching device to improve mandibular mobility after composite resection: a pilot study. Arch Phys Med Rehabil 2005;86(7):1416–9.
43. Shulman DH, Shipman B, Willis FB. Treating trismus with dynamic splinting: a cohort, case series. Adv Ther 2008;25(1):9–15.
44. Langmore SE, Terpenning MS, Schork A, et al. Predictors of aspiration pneumonia: how important is dysphagia? Dysphagia 1998;13(2):69–81.
45. Terpenning MS, Taylor GW, Lopatin DE, et al. Aspiration pneumonia: dental and oral risk factors in an older veteran population. J Am Geriatr Soc 2001;49(5):557–63.
46. Dirix P, Nuyts S, Van den Bogaert W. Radiation-induced xerostomia in patient with head and neck cancer: a literature review. Cancer 2006;107(11):2525–34.
47. De Boer MF, McCormick LK, Pruyn JF, et al. Physical and psychosocial correlates of head and neck cancer: a review of the literature. Otolaryngol Head Neck Surg 1999;120(3):427–36.
48. Kulbersh BD, Rosenthal EL, McGrew BM, et al. Pretreatment, preoperative swallowing exercises may improve dysphagia quality of life. Laryngoscope 2006; 116(6):883–6.
49. Carroll WR, Locher JL, Canon CL, et al. Pretreatment swallowing exercises improve swallow function after chemoradiation. Laryngoscope 2008;118(1):39–43.
50. Sackett DL, Straus SE, Richardson WS, et al. Evidence-based medicine: how to practice and teach EBM. Edinburgh (United Kingdom): Churchill Livingstone; 2000.

51. Clark HM. Neuromuscular treatments for speech and swallowing. Am J Speech Lang Pathol 2003;12(4):400–15.
52. Kupferman ME, Acevedo J, Hutcheson KA, et al. Addressing an unmet need in oncology patients: rehabilitation of upper aerodigestive tract function. Ann Oncol 2011;22(10):2299–303.

The Psychosocial Care Needs of Patients with HPV-Related Head and Neck Cancer

Dorothy Gold, MSW, LCSW-C, OSW-C

KEYWORDS

- Head and neck cancer • HPV-psychosocial distress • Symptom burden
- Depression • Anxiety • Quality of life • Psychosocial needs • Support services
- Oncology social work

KEY POINTS

- A diagnosis of head and neck cancer (HNC) can be devastating because of feelings of shock, uncertainty and a fear of disfigurement, dysfunction, or disability.
- Patients with HNC confront physical and psychosocial challenges throughout the disease trajectory.
- There exists a high potential for psychosocial distress, including anxiety and depression, throughout the continuum of care, including survivorship.
- Patients with human papillomavirus (HPV)-related HNC are at increased risk for emotional distress because of their demographic profile as well as the viral cause of their tumors.
- Unmet psychosocial needs can complicate the course of treatment and recovery.
- There is a need for psychosocial assessment and support services for patients with HNC, including the subset of patients with HPV-related HNC, which in turn can maximize adjustment and quality of life.

Abbreviations: PSYCHOSOCIAL CARE NEEDS OF HEAD & NECK CANCER PATIENTS	
HNC	Head and neck cancer
HNSCC	Head and neck squamous cell carcinoma
HPV-HNC	Human papilloma virus-related head & neck cancer
QOL	Quality of life

INTRODUCTION

The moment a person learns that they have cancer, the person feels as though the world has suddenly stopped and a storm of emotions sweeps in to fill the void.

Disclosure: Nothing to disclose.
Milton J. Dance, Jr. Head and Neck Center, Greater Baltimore Medical Center (GBMC), 6569 North Charles Street, Suite 401, Baltimore, MD 21204, USA
E-mail address: dgold@gbmc.org

Otolaryngol Clin N Am 45 (2012) 879–897
doi:10.1016/j.otc.2012.05.001   oto.theclinics.com
0030-6665/12/$ – see front matter © 2012 Elsevier Inc. All rights reserved.

Disbelief, shock, anxiety, and fear are among those feelings. The realization that it is a head and neck cancer (HNC) intensifies the reaction because of the proximity of the cancer site to the vital structures important to breathing, speaking, chewing, and swallowing. There is not only a fear of death but also of a survival threatened with disability, disfigurement, and dysfunction.

Confusion compounds the shock when the person receiving the diagnosis is young, active, otherwise healthy, and possesses none of the classic risk factors such as extensive tobacco or alcohol abuse. This is the picture of the patient likely to receive a diagnosis of the unique subset of head and neck squamous cell carcinoma (HNSCC) that is associated with human papillomavirus (HPV).[1] The mix of emotions that erupt on that day begins a journey marked by physical and psychosocial stresses. Those facing an HPV-related HNC (HPV-HNC), like the broader group of patients with HNC, confront physical and psychological challenges associated with diagnosis and treatment. In addition, this group face anxieties related to the cause and transmission of HPV, an aspect of patient care that has been underappreciated but that can confound adjustment. Furthermore, there are individual strengths and obstacles for each patient that play a role during the disease trajectory.

Patients with oropharyngeal HNC experience disproportionate psychosocial distress both at baseline and as a consequence of the disease. Most persons with HNC have a history of significant tobacco use; many also report heavy alcohol use. Some patients experience depressive symptoms even before a diagnosis is made,[2] although others are likely to develop depression after treatment.[3]

Surgical options cause facial disfigurement, which is usually visible. Organ preservation can now be achieved through combined chemotherapy and radiation regimens as the primary treatment. This strategy has provided promise and improved survival rates, but not without cost. Even when treatment is curative, concern about short-term and long-term quality of life (QOL) can be a factor in recovery because of the severe treatment-related toxicities.[4] These side effects, like the disease itself, strike at the primary areas of daily functioning that are normally taken for granted, such as eating, speaking, and breathing. Thus, there is a threat to the basic elements of QOL at diagnosis, during treatment, and throughout survivorship.

Psychosocial distress has been associated with all cancers, but particularly with HNCs. In site-specific comparisons, HNC is among those groups experiencing the highest levels of distress as measured within 90 days of diagnosis.[5] Likewise, depression measured independently is prevalent in many oncology patients. Within specific cancer groups, patients with HNC, and predominantly those with oropharyngeal cancers, experience the highest rates of major depressive disorder, (22%–57%).[6] HNC creates challenges because of the nature of the tumor site, the possible impact on facial appearance and function, and the symptom burden resulting from treatment. There exists a high potential for depression and general distress.

There is scarce research dedicated to psychosocial distress in the subset of HPV-HNC. However, there are reasons to suggest that this subset may be at high risk. These cancers are primarily oropharyngeal,[7] a tumor site that has been associated with high rates of depression. Patients are more likely to undergo the combined modality treatments[8] that produce many adverse affects. Moreover, HPV-related cancers are known to be sexually transmitted and have been correlated with specific sexual behavior patterns, including a high number of partners, young age of first sexual encounter, high frequency of oral sex, and marijuana use.[9,10] The relationship between sexual behavior and HPV-related oropharyngeal cancers can further contribute to emotional turmoil and depression.[11] The acknowledgment that one's cancer is derived from a sexually transmitted infection can be a source of distress.

Psychosocial factors and distress can have a far-reaching impact on QOL and adjustment at all points in the disease trajectory. Accordingly, it is important to understand the variables that constitute QOL and their relationship to psychosocial adjustment. This understanding provides the framework to describe and understand the psychosocial factors and challenges that face patients with HNC, including those with HPV-related tumors, as they journey through the course of their disease from diagnosis, treatment, and recovery to survivorship.

QOL AND PSYCHOSOCIAL ADJUSTMENT
What is QOL?

The World Health Organization defines QOL as "a state of complete physical, mental, and social well-being, and not merely the absence of disease or infirmity."[12] Traditionally, treatment success has been measured by tumor reduction or disease-free survival.[13] Advances in treatment of HNC have generated multiple treatment options with equal disease-free outcomes. There has also been acknowledgment that there are substantial late effects of combined modality treatment.[14] Consequently, new emphasis has been placed on QOL and psychosocial adjustment to both disease and its treatment.[15] The question is not so much "Can this cure me?" but rather "Can this cure me and how will it leave me?" or "What will my life be like when I am done?" These are legitimate questions that should be considered in the treatment planning stage.

QOL encompasses multiple dimensions beyond physical health and well-being:

- It may be measured in part by number or intensity of physical symptoms.
- QOL incorporates social and psychological well-being and includes such key elements as:
  - Satisfaction with home life
  - Satisfaction with family
  - Satisfaction with religion
  - Satisfaction with education or income
  - Ability to work
  - Daily functional activities, including eating and speaking.

The increasing cohort of patients with HPV-related oropharyngeal cancers will no doubt place greater emphasis on these broader areas of living. The trend for better disease outcomes in this group,[8,16] coupled with a younger age of onset,[7] presumes a long survivorship. Thus, survivors need to address the psychosocial stressors and adaptive challenges that may result from various treatments over a long period.

How is QOL Measured?

Measuring these areas is difficult because they can be based on a subjective perception of satisfaction. The World Health Organization further explains QOL as "an individual's perception of their position in life, in the context of the culture and value systems in their life and in relation to their goals, expectations, standards, and concerns."[17] This perception can create differing assumptions between patient, family, or health care providers. In addition, there is the added dimension of community manifested by societal expectations and interpretations of the patient's QOL. Thus, there may be a discrepancy in which:

- A patient may report feeling fine, but family members may think that the patient is not eating enough or trying hard enough.
- A physician may report that a patient is doing well, whereas the same patient may say or think that they are "a mess".

- A patient may feel too embarrassed to go out with friends, although friends are proud of the strength and courage of the patient and want to make social plans.
- The patient's subjective experience can vary and not be associated consistently with functional outcomes.[18]
- Patients can score high on QOL scores but report significant depression, or have poor functional scores but minimal depressive symptoms.

It is not clear from research why these discrepancies occur, but it is an area that continues to be studied.[19] Understanding and interpreting QOL can be a complex process. Yet, in the setting of multiple treatment choices, these variables carry greater weight as one means of determining an optimal regimen.

Which QOL Instruments are Used in HNC Research?

Many QOL instruments are used in HNC research,[20] including:

1. University of Washington[21]
2. EORTC (European Organisation for Research and Treatment of Cancer) 30 and 35[22]
3. FACT-HN (Functional Assessment of Cancer Therapy–Head and Neck).[23]

These 3 questionnaires cover multiple domains, including:

- Functional
- Emotional
- Social
- Subset of HNC-specific questions.

Other surveys measure depression and anxiety independently. Frequently used instruments include inventories created for the general population:

1. HADS (Hospital Anxiety and Depression Survey)[24]
2. Beck Depression Scale[25]
3. BSI (Brief Symptom Inventory).[26]

Some studies compare elements of QOL measures with depression or anxiety measures as a way to understand the interrelationships.[19] These instruments are each based on patient self-report and provide the patient's subjective analysis of the situation.

How Do Psychosocial Factors Affect QOL Appraisal?

Psychosocial factors can play an important role in influencing the subjective elements of one's personal appraisal of QOL. Likewise, psychosocial challenges and how they are managed can play a significant role in adjustment and in QOL. These challenges may:

- Present at time of diagnosis, preexisting
- Present at time of diagnosis, as a result of the diagnosis and impending treatment
- Develop and change during treatment, and throughout recovery and survivorship.

Examining the psychosocial challenges throughout this continuum of care enhances understanding of adjustment and QOL. Specifically, 4 stages are explored:

1. Diagnosis
2. Treatment
3. Recovery
4. Long-term survivorship.

The unique challenges and responses of each phase are described, along with possible interventions. Current research on psychological distress and coping during treatment is general to most HNC types and may distinguish between tumor subsets and treatment modalities. There is negligible research that explores the psychosocial challenges and needs specific to the cohort of HPV-HNC. However, available HNC research, theory, and clinical experience provide insight in to the needs of this group. In light of their increasing numbers, a new impetus to investigate their unique psychosocial construct is warranted.

DIAGNOSIS STAGE OF HNC

The diagnostic stage can be considered the period that begins with the onset of symptoms and continues through the diagnosis and treatment planning phase. When people are first confronted with symptoms that are merely suspicious for cancer, they begin to feel anxiety and turmoil. Jimmie Holland MD in her book *The Human Side of Cancer* describes this phenomenon, noting the emotions evoked by the initial fear of a cancer diagnosis and then magnified by its confirmation. These emotions include anxiety, shock, disbelief, fear, and uncertainty about the future. People who have never contemplated their own death are suddenly confronted with the realization, "I can die from this."[27] This reaction is compounded for the patient with HNC by added fears of dysfunction and disfigurement. Many people have preconceived notions of what treatment of HNC entails. They have images of disfigured faces and incomprehensible speech. Younger patients, as commonly associated with HPV-HNC, are likely active, healthy, employed, and socially involved, potentially leading to a greater sense of shock and confusion. Younger patients also have younger families, which generates fears about providing for or even being there for their family. The shock of this diagnosis is further colored by the realization that HPV is a sexually transmitted infection. This realization spawns fear of stigma, feelings of guilt or doubt, and questions for partners and spouses about sexual history.

Short Interval from Diagnosis to Treatment Planning

There is little time to absorb the shock of the diagnosis because patient and family quickly enter the treatment planning stage. For the patient with HNC, this involves:

- A myriad of appointments with specialists
- A potentially prolonged interval between the onset of symptoms, diagnosis, and treatment planning
- Conflicting information complicated by the Internet
- The prospect of an uncertain future.

The result can be any combination of depression, frustration, anxiety, annoyance, confusion, and fear. Patients often describe the period from diagnosis to start of treatment as the worst time in their disease.[27] When considering a typical scenario for a patient with newly diagnosed HNC and in particular one with an HPV-related diagnosis, it is easy to comprehend the complexity of this period.

Effect of Symptoms

Symptoms of HNC are often insidious, which delays a definitive diagnosis.

- Patients often start with 1 or several medical professionals, including a primary care physician, dentist, or general otolaryngologist before reaching an HNC specialist.
- They may have been given 1 or 2 courses of antibiotics before undergoing a biopsy.

- In the case of a younger patient presenting without the classic risk factors, particularly significant tobacco or alcohol abuse, a suspicion of cancer is not high in a differential diagnosis list.
- Anxiety and fear can build up during this period of uncertainty and continued symptoms.
- This period can last from weeks to months.

Diagnosis Confirmation

- When the diagnosis is finally confirmed, patients and families may experience anger or guilt.
- The diagnosis itself creates turmoil and crisis marked by a range of strong emotions beginning with disbelief, and high anxiety.
- As the reality of the situation sets in, there are feelings of dysphoria marked by further anxiety, depression, poor concentration, and difficulty sleeping.
- It may be difficult to process all of the information.
- There is adaptation to the diagnosis and treatment.[28]

A patient typically moves from disbelief to dysphoria and adaptation quickly, often in a matter of weeks. At the same time, the patients and families must continue to manage and coordinate additional medical appointments along with important treatment decisions.

Transition from Diagnosis to Treatment

The patient with newly diagnosed HNC is confronted with many disease-related demands as they move to treatment.

- The demands evoke feelings of confusion, impatience, and fears for consequences of delays in treatment.
- Patients and families are introduced to new concepts such as feeding tubes, port catheters, fluoride trays, and radiation masks. Previously unknown, these medical devices are soon to be part of their day-to-day living.
- When radiation is part of the treatment plan, the patient with HNC also must undergo a fitting for the face mask; that alone can be a traumatic experience, especially for someone who is claustrophobic.
- Patients must then embrace the reality that this mask will be placed on them for every radiation treatment, that the feeding tube may become the primary source of nutrition, and that their lives will be controlled by treatment schedules.

Patterns of Anxiety and Depression

Dealing with these tumultuous emotions is demanding. Managing these feelings along with the challenges of this early period is different for each individual. Each patient brings unique life experiences as well as physical and psychological morbidities as they confront diagnosis.

- Many patients with HNC have preexisting mental health problems, such as depression, anxiety, alcohol or tobacco abuse, or cognitive decline related to age or addiction.[29]
- Patients with HNC have been shown to have a higher incidence of depression and suicide compared with the general cancer population.[30] Davies and colleagues[2] examined depression among patients with HNC in the investigative stage. Patients awaiting biopsy results completed depression surveys; findings showed that a positive biopsy result was correlated with a higher incidence of prediagnosis depression.

- Patients with no previous history of mental health problems have also been known to develop new-onset depression after diagnosis, most likely as a reaction to their cancer.[31]

These patterns are significant because research has shown that psychosocial distress at baseline is a predictor of problems during and after cancer treatment.

- Howren and colleagues[32] found that even the presence of mild depressive symptoms before the start of treatment can have a significant deleterious effect on health-related QOL, including eating and swallowing.
- Pretreatment depression has been correlated with higher levels of posttreatment depression.[33–36] In 1 study, depression was identified as a strong but modifiable risk factor for malnutrition in patients undergoing radiotherapy for HNC.[37]
- Preexisting anxiety has also been correlated with posttreatment anxiety.[34,37]
- In addition to morbidities, certain demographic variables are associated with depression and anxiety[31]:
  o Employment status (working at the time of cancer diagnosis)
  o Younger age (<55 years)
  o Single marital status
  o Living alone
- Several studies have concluded that anxiety is more prevalent in younger patients.[38]
- Male patients are more likely to have posttreatment anxiety.[34]

The demographics of young age, male, and active involvement in careers characterize the HPV-HNC population, suggesting they may be at higher risk for depression and anxiety.

Coping Styles

Coping styles have also been shown to influence disease adjustment and outcome.

- In 1 study, deniers and fighters were noted to have significantly more favorable management of their illness[39]:
  o The denier minimizes the illness, shows little emotional expression, but compliantly completes all treatment demands
  o The fighter displays excessive emotion, even aggressiveness, and remains involved and active in their treatment
- Verdonck-de Leeuw and colleagues[40] reported that a passive coping style in patients and spouses correlated with greater distress.

This range of morbidities and personal variables accompany patients as they face their diagnosis and treatment, which then interplay with the medical treatment regimen and can influence outcome.

Comorbidities

As patients approach treatment, they must confront their history of emotional difficulties or substance abuse.

Psychiatric problems
Patients with significant psychiatric problems may require a pretreatment evaluation with acute intervention. The newer aggressive treatment regimens require physical, psychological, and social strength.[41]

Tobacco and alcohol use

Tobacco and alcohol abuse should also be addressed at this time. It is particularly critical to address alcohol abuse for surgical patients because of the risk for a complicated alcohol withdrawal and prolonged hospitalization. Nicotine can also negatively affect healing and postsurgical complications. Continued nicotine use also places patients at higher risk of recurrence.[42] A portion of HPV-positive patients also have a history of heavy tobacco or alcohol use.[10] Accordingly, these variables should not be ignored in the HPV-positive group.

Sexually transmitted disease

The subset of younger patients with HPV-related HNSCC may present with high levels of anxiety because of the unexpectedness of the diagnosis, their fears related to the consequences of the disease on their young families, and the realization that their cancer derives from a sexually transmitted infection. In addition to fears and adjustment to a cancer diagnosis, patients must confront the implications of the correlation of their cancer to HPV. They must deal with their own reaction as well as that of their partner, their family, and their community.

A review of literature on HPV testing and cervical screenings for women can provide insight into the range and extent of emotions possible when dealing with a sexually transmitted disease:

- Research on HPV testing for women as part of cervical cancer screening has suggested that an HPV-positive result may have an adverse psychosocial impact for the women tested, with increased anxiety, distress, and concern about sexual relationships.[43]
- A qualitative study of the impact of repeated HPV testing on women that included in-depth interviews reported that feelings of shock, confusion, and distress about testing HPV-positive were common for these women.
- Emotions were commonly related to concerns about sexual transmission, the cause of the virus, and anxiety about the health implications.
- A lack of knowledge about HPV seemed to trigger anxiety, often leading to frantic Internet searches to answer questions that may arise.[44]
- Similarly, patients confronted with an oropharyngeal HPV-associated malignancy can experience anxiety and distress as they try to understand the implications of HPV infection and its connection to their cancer.
- There may be questions about cause that can lead to concerns about fidelity, past relations, and underlying suspicions by the spouse.

These variables can potentiate stress in a relationship already burdened by the strain of the cancer itself at a time that adaptation to treatment is critical. Patients and their partners require reliable and comprehensible information from the health care team so that these issues can be addressed.

Social and financial support

Patients with HNC may also present with either inadequate or no family, social, financial, or health insurance support. These variables can affect treatment compliance and adjustment.[45]

- Living alone and having no spouse or partner have been correlated with delay in seeking treatment[46] and have been determined to be predictors of psychological distress for newly diagnosed patients with HNC.[47]
- Financial worries can contribute to additional stress for patient and family. This stress can be equally applicable to patients diagnosed with an HPV-HNC despite

their tendency to be of higher socioeconomic status. Often, families must work hard to maintain a high standard of living, including overtime, second jobs, and debt; as a result, there can be a fear of losing a portion of income essential to paying bills and maintaining lifestyle. Likewise, decisions about health insurance coverage may have been made based on costs, leaving a risk of high deductibles or medical copayments or even having no insurance.

The knowledge that psychosocial factors present at diagnosis can have far-reaching impact beyond the treatment stage underscores the need for a psychosocial assessment to be part of the initial workup. Preexisting psychosocial concerns and problems can be addressed early with appropriate information and referrals and then followed by ongoing support. This strategy can enhance adjustment and successful management of aggressive treatment choices.

PSYCHOSOCIAL FACTORS DURING THE TREATMENT STAGE

Once the diagnosis is made and a treatment plan is developed, the patient enters the treatment phase, often bringing with them unresolved emotions and fears. Treatment may involve radiation only, surgery alone, surgery followed by adjuvant therapies, or concurrent chemoradiation as primary treatment. There are challenges inherent in each treatment choice.

Surgery

The surgical patient may need to deal with the resulting disfigurement and dysfunction. A patient may have a tracheostomy or feeding tube; may have lost their larynx, or part of their tongue. These are major life changes that also require new learning regarding self-care, speaking, or swallowing.

Radiation

Primary surgery is often followed by adjuvant therapies, either radiation alone or combined with chemotherapy. Pain, dysgeusia, mucositis, difficulty swallowing, nausea, fatigue, and other troublesome side effects accompany these treatments.

Combined Treatments

Aggressive combined modality regimens as the primary treatment may avoid major disfiguring surgery but produce more adverse effects and intensified physical complaints.[41] These symptoms can also contribute to complex emotional responses such as anxiety, irritability, frustration, disgust, depression, anger, and family strain.[48]

Depression and Anxiety

Research has supported the strong prevalence of depression and anxiety in patients undergoing treatments for HNC. Kelly and colleagues[36] found that depression increased during the course of treatment with decrement in QOL, peaking at the end of treatment. These investigators determined that up to 24.2% of the patients were depressed before treatment, but even patients who started treatment without depression showed a tendency to become depressed as treatment progressed. Conversely, anxiety seemed to be higher at the start of treatment but diminished over time. These investigators also determined that the addition of chemotherapy to the treatment program was associated with higher levels of posttreatment depression. Nelson and colleagues[34] reported similar trends. Depressive symptoms intensified, whereas QOL worsened during the course of radiotherapy and was worse for patients also receiving chemotherapy. Similarly, anxiety became less significant during the same period. In addition, patients treated with aggressive hyperfractionated radiation therapy have been reported to be at higher risk for depression.[49]

Many studies have investigated the prevalence and patterns of distress and depression for this group of patients, identifying a host of associated variables that some studies support or others contradict. However, there is sufficient evidence to conclude that treatments for HNC in general are associated with psychosocial distress, including anxiety and depression. Moreover, it is likely that the subset of patients with HPV-related diagnosis may be at particular risk, given that they are mostly young men with oropharyngeal malignancies who undergo multimodality treatment that can include chemotherapy and possibly hyperfractionated radiation as part of their regimen.

Social and Economic Adjustments

Social and economic factors also come into play during the treatment period for patient and family. Job security, adequate sick leave, health care coverage, and disability benefits, as well as income loss, can generate stress, create anxiety, and affect adjustment. Administrative forms required by employers or insurance companies may seem overwhelming. The self-employed may fear missing work for an extended period because of concern about loss of income or the viability of their business. Unrealistic expectations about continuing routine activities during treatment may arise, later met with despair when they cannot be achieved.

Family Stress

The treatment phase can also be trying for the family and larger support network because of feelings of helplessness in the context of personal turmoil.[50] Gotay[51] identified a range of fears experienced by family members, including the fear of the cancer diagnosis, future ability to perform family functions, general emotional disturbances, the effect of illness on employment, the possibility of a terminal illness, restrictions on activities, side effects of treatment, and concern about the family's future. Simultaneously, families must establish new routines. Disease and treatment must be incorporated into day-to-day living. Ordinary responsibilities do not disappear and balancing these competing demands can amplify stress. Spouses or other family members want to be available for support, but worry about their own jobs or their children's needs. The disease and treatment can become a life intrusion because it disrupts daily routines and creates stress. By the nature of their demographic factors, patients with HPV-HNC, along with their families, are likely to deal with issues of family schedules, employment, finances, and general life intrusions caused by the illness and treatment. Furthermore, these younger families need to be able to talk to their children about a parent's cancer diagnosis and need to worry about ramifications with school issues. Family dynamics can be further complicated by the presence of parents/grandparents, who may be willing and able to provide help but whose own emotions are added to an already highly charged environment.

Thus, spouses and other family members need support as they deal with their own emotional response along with the stresses of caregiving. Verdonck-de Leeuw and colleagues[40] investigated the incidence of distress in spouses and patients after treatment of HNC. They recorded a clinical level of distress in 20% of spouses, and determined that high distress was related to the presence of a feeding tube in patients, a passive coping style, less vitality, and a disrupted daily life schedule from caregiving. In addition, the spouses of patients with malignancies of the larynx and oral/oropharynx reported higher scores of distress compared with those with parotid tumors. The results also identified a tendency for higher distress scores among spouses of patients treated with chemoradiation. These findings support the probability of greater anxiety among spouses of patients with HPV-HNC. These younger spouses, usually wives, must deal with their own fears and concerns for the patient and also manage the children and handle role reversal with regard to family responsibilities. The ability to identify patients/families at high risk and to provide psychosocial support can enhance adjustment.

Psychosocial Interventions

Interventions to assist during the treatment phase include psychoeducation, information and referrals to helpful resources, medications for pain, anxiety, and depression, as well as assistance with problem solving and basic emotional support. Relaxation exercises can provide a tool for patients and their families to manage their emotions. Talking to other patients, especially someone who has successfully completed similar treatment, can provide immense encouragement, especially during the rough times during treatment. There are also many online resources that help patients and families share information and organize volunteers who can provide practical assistance. Such tools can be especially helpful to young families dealing with aggressive multimodality treatments.

Thus, anxiety levels may diminish during the treatment phase as questions are answered and there is active involvement in a plan to do something for the cancer. However, the treatment stage also brings new challenges that include the burden of physical symptoms, as well as family, financial, employment, and health coverage concerns. Patients must deal with a deteriorating QOL and the risk of increased distress and depression. They must also be able to successfully complete treatment.

RECOVERY

Patients, families, and members of the health care team express joy and relief when treatment comes to an end. However, the adverse effects do not cease immediately after the end of treatment. Patients should be prepared for this reality. Yet even when counseled, patients can experience distress and disappointment when recovery is neither immediate nor fast.

Early Recovery Period

Sherman and colleagues,[48] in their research on coping with HNC during different phases of treatment, reported increased distress and significant use of coping mechanisms in the immediate aftermath of treatment, suggesting that this may be a particularly demanding period. This situation may be explained by the sudden loss of attention and activity, which is in stark contrast to the active treatment phase, with daily treatments, multiple appointments, and frequent encounters with different members of the health care team. Treatment sequelae are at their peak and do not begin to improve immediately. Simultaneously, financial, work, and family issues must be handled. Patients who are on short-term disability plan their return to work. They may be pulled by a sense of urgency to return when physically they are not ready.

Comparison of Different Recovery Periods

The incidence of depression has been determined as highest at the end of treatment but can continue to linger during recovery.

- Katz and colleagues[52] studied depression in patients 1 month after completion of radiotherapy and found that a significant minority of patients report depression 1 month after completing treatment.

- Kelly and colleagues[36] reported depression as still prevalent at 3 months and 6 months after treatment and start to show a slow return to pretreatment levels at about 12 months. Furthermore, the investigators considered their findings as underestimations, assuming that depressed patients were more likely to drop out of the study.

This latter pattern supports an earlier study that measured psychological distress at 6 time points during 1 year: time of diagnosis and then 1, 2, 3, 6, and 12 months after treatment. Close to one-third of patients were found to have a possible or probable mood disorder at each of the time points. In addition, new cases of anxiety or depression were identified at each time point. Anxiety was determined as higher at time of diagnosis, whereas depression seemed to be highest during treatment.[53] Thus, depression and psychological distress:

- Can be preexisting problems for the patient
- Can present at time of diagnosis as a reaction to the illness
- Can increase or originate at different points throughout treatment
- Are likely to be present in the early months after treatment ends
- Can potentially onset anew after treatment ends and during recovery.

These findings highlight the need for supportive care and psychological counseling during the early recovery period. Likewise, the health care team should be alert to the potential for distress after treatment ends and be prepared to assess for this at routine follow-up visits, allowing for timely and appropriate referrals.

Psychosocial Education

Patients and families must be prepared for recovery. They should be educated about the physical and emotional symptoms that may be experienced. There should be an understanding of what to expect and how to manage such symptoms, along with a path of action for unmanageable problems. There is joy when the last treatment ends. However, as patient and loved ones leave the building, they are leaving a safe place, filled with knowledgeable professionals who have provided care and attention. They are walking out into a great unknown, a place where even the well-adjusted and supported patient can become overwhelmed and stressed.

Questions, concerns, doubts, and fears about sexual behavior can resurface during recovery and during the transition to long-term survivorship. The initial shock and confusion about sexual transmission is often put aside by patients and loved ones as they become preoccupied with the demands of treatment. It is further tempered by the news of improved outcomes for HPV-HNC. However, as thoughts return to normalizing life again, it is natural for questions about HPV transmission, and return to intimacy, to arise. Emotions that may have been suppressed in order to focus on treatment can also reemerge and create tension within the relationship. It is necessary to further clarify information about oral HPV transmission, as well as to deal with any resulting emotional conflict, thereby promoting better adjustment during recovery and moving forward.

Information about resources for counseling and support should be available to patients at the end of treatment. Direct interventions at this time may include referrals for rehabilitative services, such as speech and swallowing therapy, lymphedema treatment, or physical therapy, as well as nutrition services, individual counseling, and support groups. The period directly after treatment is also stressful for the spouse or caregiver, and continued support should be made available to them as well. There has been recent emphasis on the development of a written treatment summary and survivorship plan of care that documents the patient's cancer experience and provides guidance for future care to be provided at the end of treatments, as recommended by the Institute of Medicine (IOM). It should include a treatment summary, a listing of potential long-term or late effects, a plan for ongoing medical follow- up, and links for appropriate resources.[54] This information, provided in a structured format, can reduce anxiety during recovery and better prepare patients for survivorship.

LONG-TERM SURVIVORSHIP

After recovery, the patient must begin to deal with the day-to-day issues related to long-term survivorship or simply the return to normal living. Several phases may be confronted during survivorship:

- Reintegration into normal life activities
- Adaptation to a new normal
- Dealing with fear of or actual recurrence
- Metastasis
- End-of-life care.

The survivor reintegrates to normal life activities through actions such as returning to a regular work schedule, enjoying family and social events, participating in physical activity and exercise schedules, and again enjoying events that include food. As patients are reintegrated, there needs to be acknowledgment and acceptance that there may be a new normal. The patient with HNC may need to adapt to late effects of treatment, to new dietary or swallowing restrictions, or to an altered appearance. Patients and partners need to understand and be comfortable with the implications of the sexual transmission of HPV. Moreover, patients who had been treated for HPV-related malignancies are more likely to have to confront work, financial, and family matters, even as their bodies are rebuilding.

Common Concerns for Cancer Survivors

Common concerns for cancer survivors in general have been identified as[28]:

- Fear of recurrence
- Worry about delayed physical effects
- Risk of second cancers
- A sense of uncertainty about the future
- A greater sense of vulnerability.

The fear of recurrence or second cancers can be pervasive, especially when young families are involved. Thus, minor physical symptoms may be feared as signs of recurrent cancer. Likewise, anxiety and panic may develop before follow-up appointments or diagnostic tests. Younger patients with greater family responsibility could experience this anxiety with greater force.

Depression in Cancer Survivors

There remains a continued concern for depression during survivorship. Murphy and colleagues[14] point to a qualitative study that assessed impact of HNC on patients and caregivers. Several important themes were identified in the aftermath of treatment, including:

- Fear of recurrence
- Role transitions in family and work

- Dealing with lingering side effects
- Mood disorders.

There is evidence that depression can be present up to 6 years after diagnosis.[40] Moreover, there are some data indicating that the greatest improvement in mental distress in patients with HNC occurs 3 years after treatment compared with other QOL domains.[55] These patterns underline the need for ongoing attention to psychosocial factors, as well as making supportive care and counseling services available for several years after diagnosis.

Cancer Recurrence

Some survivors face cancer again. Even with the improved outcome rates noted for HPV-HNCs, some patients face recurrence, metastatic disease, or new primary cancers. Emotions notable at initial diagnosis reappear more powerfully and may hinder the ability to adapt to this new reality. It becomes difficult to maintain a positive attitude the second time around as patients and loved ones grapple with the larger, often unanswerable, question of "Why?" This situation can be particularly difficult for patients with HPV-related cancers who were advised about a better prognosis. At this time, new choices and decisions are confronted as treatment options are explored.[56] Salvage surgeries can be more complex and result in greater disability. Other therapies carry further risk for toxicities. There is heightened concern about functional consequences in terms of breathing, eating, and swallowing. There are also many confusing choices for treatment in the ever-increasing options for advanced recurrent or metastatic HNC. Some may be driven to search for the best option, now simplified by the Internet. These scenarios can produce a jumble of emotions that range from hope and fight to fatigue and fear and that lead to personal and family stress. Side effects and morbidities continue to retain importance with any treatment choices. In those instances in which progression of illness occurs, there is a corresponding fear of pain, as well as a fear of losing the ability to eat and speak. It is important for the health care team to acknowledge that these fears exist, to address them, and to assist with realistic planning. The burden and the benefit of each treatment should be considered. Ideally, questions about advanced directives, health care proxy, and resuscitation wishes should be addressed early in the disease process before any medical crisis might occur. It is important for surgeons and oncologists to be comfortable discussing these topics with patients and caregivers and to ensure that they are handled in a timely fashion.

End-of-Life Issues

In the face of advanced disease, end-of-life issues enter the picture.[56] For many, the search for ongoing treatment continues relentlessly, even as the body weakens. The question of when to stop has been described as "the elephant in the room."[57] For some patients and families, the decision to stop treatment can be more difficult than deciding which type of primary or secondary treatment to receive. The treatment team needs to ensure that they are providing adequate information to allow fully informed decisions regarding the choice of aggressive treatment or palliative care. At the same time, it is important to be sensitive to the patient or family's emotional state and their readiness for this discussion. This can be a difficult balance. Some patients need to continue an improbable fight for life even in the face of suffering, whereas others focus on QOL and comfort.[57] However, the medical team needs to be compassionate and honest, so that patients and families are allowed the opportunity to understand their reality and make appropriate decisions.

As end of life nears, it may be necessary to deal with critical decisions about pain, airway management, swallowing, and maintaining nutrition.[58] This situation can create tension and controversy with patient, family, and health care professionals. Management of symptoms and functional deficits at this point can be complicated by the unique qualities of the disease coupled with the organs affected. Inability to eat can be a result of tumor obstruction or a manifestation of the end-of-life process. Decisions about tracheotomies and feeding tubes with progressive disease can be delicate, and need to be made with full consideration to goals of care. For an older patient or one who lives alone with little social support, these procedures may solve an immediate symptom, but may determine whether a patient can remain independent in the community or require skilled nursing placement. On the other hand, a younger or well-supported patient may experience a better QOL with the addition of a tracheotomy or a feeding tube even when their disease is life-limiting. These can be difficult decisions; patients look to the health care team for honest guidance, and decisions should not be made from medical science alone but instead with consideration to the psychosocial considerations of the patient and the family.

Table 1
Psychosocial care needs at different stages of the disease

Stage	Emotional/Life Stress Points	Psychosocial Needs
Diagnosis	Shock, disbelief, fear of uncertain future	Psychosocial assessment
	Dysphoria, depression, anxiety	Coping with emotions
	Information overload, overwhelmed	Education about illness, treatment,
	Confusion	and symptom burden
	Impatience to start treatment	Guidance to navigate health care system
	Financial, work, and family stresses	Patient mentor
Treatment	Symptom burden/functional changes	Counseling for emotional support, coping skills
	QOL deterioration	Resource information and referrals
	Depression, irritability, frustration, anxiety	Psychoeducation
	Disruptions in work, family, and social life	Stress management, relaxation exercises
	Stress on the family	Psychosocial care for the family
	Financial/employment concerns	Problem solving for practical needs
Recovery	Toxicities/symptom burden at peak	Ongoing monitoring for support and guidance
	Loss of contact with health care team	Reassessment of psychosocial needs
	Discouragement with rate of recovery	Referrals to rehabilitative and support team members
	Increased distress	Address family psychosocial needs
Long-term survivorship	Reentry to normal living	Encourage physical, social activity
	Accepting new normal	Counsel readaptive changes
	Potential for ongoing or new-onset depression	Assess for depression
	Fear of recurrence	Coping strategies, stress management
	Anxiety about medical appointments	Support groups
	Dealing with recurrent, metastatic or new cancer	Psychoeducation for decision making
	End-of-life issues	Palliative care resources
		Counseling to patient and family

SUMMARY AND CHALLENGES FOR THE FUTURE

QOL factors play an important role in the survivorship experience of patients with HNC. From the moment of diagnosis and on through treatment, recovery, and long-term survivorship, the physical, emotional, spiritual, and social impacts of the disease and treatment are crucial aspects of overall health outcomes. In the face of new and diverse treatment choices, often with equal outcomes, evaluating the impact of treatment on QOL is vital (**Table 1**). The number of HPV-related oropharyngeal cancers is increasing and the need to understand the unique challenges that this population faces is important. New information continues to emerge about this subset of HNC. However, scant research exists pertaining to the key psychosocial elements of this group or their patterns of distress and depression. Clearly, this needs to receive greater attention. On initial presentation, many of these patients appear well adjusted, but this does not preclude their risk for distress. Moreover, as the relationship between sexual behavior and oral HPV malignancies gains further recognition, the unique sexual, psychological, and social issues encountered demand greater attention.

This is a cohort of patients who are younger, primary breadwinners, and heads of households, who have younger, primarily school-aged children. They will undoubtedly live longer in the survivor role. This situation drives an emphasis on treatment choices that maximize survival and minimize symptom burden. Furthermore, there is a potential for psychosocial distress over a long period. Early identification and intervention for such distress can maximize healthy adjustment. Little is known about the long-term survivorship of patients with HPV-HNC. As these younger patients with HPV-HNC age, their patterns of late effects of treatment and recurring, metastatic or new cancers will emerge. Consequently, there is a need to compile information about their survivorship as well as the associated psychosocial and psychological challenges. This strategy would allow more effective planning for necessary psychosocial support.

The challenge for the health care team is to incorporate psychosocial assessment and services through the entire continuum of care. There is ample literature describing the multidisciplinary approach to HNC treatment, yet oncology social workers are infrequently listed among the primary disciplines. However, oncology social workers are uniquely qualified to provide psychosocial support. They view patients in the context of the many systems that define their lives such as self, home, work, spirituality, financial situation, and friendships. These same domains can be negatively affected by the cancer experience. Moreover, identifying and intervening with problems in these areas maximizes adjustment to diagnosis, treatment, recovery, and survivorship. For patients with HNC, with their unique concerns about basic daily functions and their high potential for emotional distress, the inclusion of psychosocial support services should be an integral part of their treatment experience. The latest IOM report, *Cancer Care for the Whole Patient: Meeting Psychosocial Needs*, supports this need. The report concludes that addressing psychosocial needs must be an integral part of quality cancer care.[59] This will be a mandated requirement for cancer care providers in 2012. To effectively meet this requirement for the increasing group of patients with HPV-HNC, it will be necessary to further understand their unique psychosocial needs.

REFERENCES

1. Marur S, D'Souza G, Westra WH, et al. HPV-associated head and neck cancer: a virus-related cancer epidemic. Lancet Oncol 2010;11(8):781–9.
2. Davies AD, Davies C, Delpo MC. Depression and anxiety in patients undergoing diagnostic investigations for head and neck cancers. Br J Psychiatry 1986;149: 491–3.

3. Duffy SA, Ronis DL, Valenstein M, et al. Depressive symptoms, smoking, drinking, and quality of life among head and neck cancer patients. Psychosomatics 2007;48:142–8.

4. Hanna E, Alexiou M, Morgan J, et al. Intensive chemoradiotherapy as a primary treatment for organ preservation in patients with advanced cancer of the head and neck. Arch Otolaryngol Head Neck Surg 2004;130:861–7.

5. Zabora J, Brintzenhofeszoc K, Curbow B, et al. The prevalence of psychologic distress by cancer site. Psychooncology 2001;10:19–28.

6. Massie MJ. Prevalence of depression in patients with cancer. J Natl Cancer Inst Monogr 2004;32:57–71.

7. Chaturvedi AK, Engels EA, Anderson WF, et al. Incidence trends for human papillomavirus-related and -unrelated oral squamous cell carcinomas in the United States. J Clin Oncol 2008;26:612–9.

8. Fakhry C, Westra WH, Li S, et al. Improved survival of patients with human papillomavirus-positive head and neck squamous cell carcinoma in a prospective clinical trial. J Natl Cancer Inst 2008;100(4):261–9.

9. D'Souza G, Agrawal Y, Halpern J, et al. Oral sexual behaviors associated with prevalent oral human papillomavirus infection. J Infect Dis 2009;199:1263–9.

10. Gillison ML, D'Souza G, Westra W, et al. Distinct risk factor profiles for human papillomavirus type 16-positive and human papillomavirus type 16-negative head and neck cancers. J Natl Cancer Inst 2008;100(6):407–20.

11. Lydiatt W, Moran J, Burke W. A review of depression in the head and neck cancer patient. Clin Adv Hematol Oncol 2009;7(6):397–413.

12. World Health Organization. Basic documents. 39th edition. Geneva (Switzerland): WHO; 1992.

13. Babin E, Sigston E, Hitier M, et al. Quality of life in head and neck cancers patients: predictive factors, functional and psychosocial outcome. Eur Arch Otorhinolaryngol 2008;265:265–70.

14. Murphy BA, Gilbert J, Cmelak A, et al. Symptom control issues and supportive care of patients with head and neck cancers. Clin Adv Hematol Oncol 2007; 5(10):807–21.

15. Terrell JE, Ronis DL, Fowler KE, et al. Clinical predictors of quality of life in patients with head and neck cancer. Arch Otolaryngol Head Neck Surg 2004; 130:401–8.

16. Gillison ML, Koch WM, Capone RB, et al. Evidence for a causal association between human papillomavirus and a subset of head and neck cancers. J Natl Cancer Inst 2000;92:709–20.

17. The WHOQOL Group. Development of the WHOQOL-BRIEF quality of life assessment. Psychol Med 1998;28:551–8.

18. Haisfield-Wolfe ME, McGuire DB, Soeken K, et al. Prevalence and correlates of depression among patients with head and neck cancer: a systematic review of implications for research. Oncol Nurs Forum 2009;36(3):E107–25.

19. List MA, Siston A, Haraf D, et al. Quality of life and performance in advanced head and neck cancer patients on concomitant chemotherapy: a prospective examination. J Clin Oncol 1999;17(3):1020–8.

20. Murphy BZ, Ridner S, Wells N, et al. Quality of life research in head and neck cancer: a review of the current state of the science. Crit Rev Oncol Hematol 2007;62:251–67.

21. Weymuller EA Jr, Alsarraf R, Yueh B, et al. Analysis of the performance characteristics of the University of Washington Quality of Life Instrument and its modification (UW-QOL-R). Arch Otolaryngol Head Neck Surg 2001;127:489–93.

22. Bjordal K, Ahlner-Elmqvist M, Tollesson E, et al. Development of a European Organisation for Research and Treatment of Cancer (EORTC) questionnaire module to be used in the quality of life assessment in head and neck cancer patients. Acta Oncol 1994;33(8):879–85.

23. D'Antonio LI, Zimmerman G, Celia DF, et al. Quality of life and functional status measures in patients with head and neck cancer. Arch Otolaryngol Head Neck Surg 1996;122:482–7.

24. Zigmond AS, Snaith RP. The hospital anxiety and depression scale. Acta Psychiatr Scand 1983;63:361–70.

25. Beck AT, Ward CH, Mendelson M, et al. An inventory for measuring depression. Arch Gen Psychiatry 1961;4:561–71.

26. Derogatis LR, Melisaratos N. The brief symptom inventory: an introductory report. Psychol Med 1983;13(3):595–605.

27. Holland JC, Lewis S. The diagnosis: "I could die of this." The human side of cancer: living with hope, coping with uncertainty. New York: Quill; 2001. p. 39–49.

28. Holland JC, Gooen-Piels JG. Principles of psycho-oncology. In: Kufe DW, Pollock RE, Holland JC, et al, editors. Cancer medicine. 5th edition. Hamilton (ON): Decker; 2000. p. 943–58.

29. McCaffrey JC, Weitzner M, Kamboukas D, et al. Alcoholism, depression and abnormal cognition in head and neck cancer: a pilot study. Otolaryngol Head Neck Surg 2007;136:92–7.

30. Zeller JL. High suicide risk found for patients with head and neck cancer. JAMA 2006;296(14):1716–7.

31. Chen AM, Jenelle RL, Grady V, et al. Prospective study of psychosocial distress among patients undergoing radiotherapy for head and neck cancer. Int J Radiat Oncol Biol Phys 2009;73(1):187–93.

32. Howren MB, Christensen AJ, Karnell LH, et al. Health-related quality of life in head and neck cancer survivors: impact of pretreatment depressive symptoms. Health Psychol 2010;29(1):65–71.

33. de Leeuw JR, de Graeff A, Ros WJ, et al. Prediction of depression 6 months to 3 years after treatment of head and neck cancer. Head Neck 2001;23:892–8.

34. Nelson KA, Pollard AC, Boonzaier AM, et al. Psychological distress (depression and anxiety) in people with head and neck cancers. Med J Aust 2010;193(5): S48–51.

35. Karnell LH, Funk GF, Christensen AJ, et al. Persistent posttreatment depressive symptoms in patients with head and neck cancer. Head Neck 2005;28: 453–61.

36. Kelly C, Paleri V, Downs C, et al. Deterioration in quality of life and depressive symptoms during radiation therapy for head and neck cancer. Otolaryngol Head Neck Surg 2007;136(1):108–11.

37. Briton B, Clover K, Bateman L, et al. Baseline depression predicts malnutrition in head and neck cancer patients undergoing radiotherapy. Support Care Cancer 2012;20(2):335–42.

38. Hutton JM, Williams M. An investigation of psychologic distress in patients who have been treated for head and neck cancer. Br J Oral Maxillofac Surg 2001; 39:333–9.

39. Greer S, Morris T, Pettingale K. Psychological response to breast cancer: effect on outcome. Lancet 1979;2(8146):785–7.

40. Verdonck-de Leeuw IM, Erenstein SE, Van der Linden MH, et al. Distress in spouses and patients after treatment for head and neck cancer. Laryngoscope 2007;117(2):238–41.

41. Murphy B, Chung C. Supportive care for patients with head and neck cancer. Medsc Hematol Oncol 2006. Available at: www.medscape.org/viewarticle541631. Accessed May 2, 2012.

42. Baile WE. Alcohol and nicotine dependency in patients with head and neck cancer. J Support Oncol 2008;6(4):165–6.

43. McCaffrey K, Waller J, Forrest S, et al. Testing positive for human papillomavirus in routine cervical screening: examination of psychosocial impact. BJOG 2004; 111(12):1437–43.

44. Waller J, McCaffery K, Kitchner H, et al. Women's experiences of repeated HPV testing in the context of cervical cancer screening: a qualitative study. Psychooncology 2007;16(3):196–204.

45. Rappaport Y, Kreitler S, Chaitchik S, et al. Psychosocial problems in head and neck cancer patients and their change with time since diagnosis. Ann Oncol 1993;4:69–73.

46. Rozniatowski O, Reich M, Mallet Y, et al. Psychosocial factors involved in delayed consultation by patients with head and neck cancer. Head Neck 2005;27(4):274–80.

47. Kugaya A, Akechi T, Okuyama T, et al. Prevalence, predictive factors, and screening for psychologic distress in patients with newly diagnosed head and neck cancer. Cancer 2000;88:2817–23.

48. Sherman AC, Simonton SC, Adams DC, et al. Coping with head and neck cancer during different phases of treatment. Head Neck 2000;22:787–93.

49. Sehlen S, Lenk M, Herschbach P, et al. Depressive symptoms during and after radiotherapy for head and neck cancer. Head Neck 2003;25:1004–18.

50. Ross S, Mosher C, Ronis-Tobin V, et al. Psychosocial adjustment of family caregivers of head and neck cancer survivors. Support Care Cancer 2010;18:171–8.

51. Gotay CC. The experience of cancer during early and advanced stages: the views of patients and their mates. Soc Sci Med 1984;18(7):605–13.

52. Katz MR, Kopek N, Waldron J, et al. Screening for depression in head and neck cancer. Psychooncology 2004;1(4):269–80.

53. Hammerlid E, Ahlner-Elmqvist M, Bjordal K, et al. A prospective multicentre study in Sweden and Norway of mental distress and psychiatric morbidity in head and neck cancer patients. Br J Cancer 1999;80:766–74.

54. Ganz PA, Hahn EE. Implementing the survivorship care plan: a strategy for improving the quality of care for cancer survivors. In: Holland JC, Breitbart WS, Jacobsen PB, et al, editors. Psycho-oncology. 2nd edition. New York: Oxford University Press; 2010. p. 557–61.

55. Hammerlid E, Silander E, Hornestam L, et al. Health-related quality of life three years after diagnosis of head and neck cancer–a longitudinal study. Head Neck 2001;23:113–25.

56. Goldstein NE, Genden E, Morrison RS. Palliative care for patients with head and neck cancer. JAMA 2008;299(15):1818–25.

57. Quill TE. Initiating end-of-life discussions with seriously ill patients. JAMA 2000; 284:2502–7.

58. Sciubba JJ. End of life considerations in the head and neck cancer patient. Oral Oncol 2009;45:431–4.

59. Holland JC, Weiss TR. The new standard of quality of cancer care in the US: the Institute of Medicine (IOM) report, cancer care for the whole patient: meeting psychosocial needs. In: Holland JC, Breitbart WS, Jacobsen PB, et al, editors. Psycho-oncology. 2nd edition. New York: Oxford University Press; 2010. p. 666–73.

Economic Impact of Human Papillomavirus–Associated Head and Neck Cancers in the United States

Diarmuid Coughlan, MPharm, MSc[a,b], Kevin D. Frick, PhD[a],*

KEYWORDS

- Economics • Cost • Economic evaluation • Human papillomavirus
- Head and neck cancer • Oropharyngeal cancer

KEY POINTS

- A literature review shows that a complete cost-of-illness study has not been conducted on head and neck cancer (HNC) in the United States.
- An *International Classification of Diseases* (ICD) code indicating the human papillomavirus (HPV) status of patients with HNC would facilitate the characterization of the economic burden of HPV-associated HNC.
- Establishing which HPV tumor-detection method in HNC is the most cost-effective would be a useful addition to clinical practice.
- The cost of treatment-related complications and patients' health-related quality of life should be factored into any cost-consequence analysis of HPV-associated HNC treatment options. Morbidity rather than mortality is the main concern in treating HPV-associated HNC.
- The increasing incidence and subsequent burden of HPV-associated HNC will be an important consideration in the HPV vaccination debate.

INTRODUCTION

The rising incidence of human papillomavirus (HPV) as the causative agent of a subset of head and neck cancers (HNC) has recently been described as an epidemic.[1–4] The reported proportion of oropharyngeal cancers attributable to HPV in the United States

Financial disclosures: The authors report no conflicts of interest.
[a] Department of Health Policy & Management, Johns Hopkins School of Public Health (JHSPH), 624 North Broadway Street, Baltimore, MD 21205, USA; [b] Department of Economics, National University of Ireland, Galway (NUIG), University Road, Galway, Ireland
* Corresponding author.
E-mail address: kfrick@jhsph.edu

Abbreviations: Economic Impact of Head and Neck Cancer			
ASCO	American Society of Clinical Oncology	LOHRAN	Longitudinal Oncology Registry of Head and Neck Carcinoma
BIA	Budget impact analysis	MEPS	Medical Expenditure Panel Survey
CDC	Centers for Disease Control and Prevention		
CEA	Cost-effectiveness analysis	MeSH	Medical Subject Heading
COI	Cost of illness	NCCN	National Comprehensive Cancer Network
CRD	Center for Reviews and Dissemination		
		NCI	National Cancer Institute
EGFR	Epidermal growth factor receptor	NHS EED	National Health Service Economic Evaluation Database (UK)
HCUP	Healthcare Cost and Utilization Project		
HNC	Head and neck cancer	PBT	Proton beam therapy
IMRT	Intensity-modulated radiation therapy	QALY	Quality adjusted life year
		QOL	Quality of life
ISPOR	International Society for Pharmacoeconomics and Outcomes Research	RT	Radiation therapy
		SEER	Surveillance, Epidemiology, and End Results
ISRCTN	International Standard Randomized Controlled Trial Number	SMDM	Society for Medical Decision Making
		TORS	Trans-oral robotic surgery

has increased from 16.3% during the 1980s to 72.7% during the 2000s.[5] More careful anatomic site stratification has made it apparent that the age-adjusted incidence of oropharyngeal cancer is rising dramatically (estimated to be a 5% annual increase).[4] In comparison with HNC not associated with HPV, incident cases of HPV-associated HNC occur primarily among younger (aged 40-59 years), nonsmoking, white men.[6,7] Hence, these virus-related cancers have been characterized in the clinical literature as being "*a distinct epidemiologic, clinical and molecular entity.*"[8]

The increasing awareness of the role of HPV in HNC in both sexes has amplified the profile of this virus even further in the public health[6,9] and mass media[10] arena. Therefore, understanding the costs of the condition is useful for making an economic argument about efforts to reduce the burden of the virus.[11] Moreover, various decision makers (providers, payers, and policy makers) will be concerned with the resulting financial impact on clinical management issues in treating such patients.[12]

The most common way to characterize the economic burden of a disease is to perform a cost-of-illness (COI) study. In this article, the components of a COI study are described. The authors then report on a literature review that was undertaken to look at the economic burden of HNC. The focus of the review was to ascertain what inferences (if any) were made about HPV. The authors elaborate on the current medical costs involved in the diagnosis, treatment, and management of these patients. Subsequently, the challenges facing the use of economic data and the controversies associated with the economic data are described, and suggestions for future research are made. The overarching aim of this article is to summarize, critique, and elaborate on the published studies that are pertinent to characterizing the economic burden of this emerging disease entity.

WHAT IS INCLUDED IN A COI STUDY?

COI studies are descriptive analyses assessing the economic burden of health problems on the population overall.[13] The traditional approach considers:

- **Direct medical costs:** Associated with emergency department and hospital services, physician services, diagnostic procedures, laboratory tests, medications, treatments, ancillary therapies, and other health care services.
- **Productivity costs:** Result from lost work productivity, disability, and premature death caused by a disease or condition.
- **Intangible costs:** Primarily related to losses in quality of life.

Together with prevalence and incidence, morbidity and mortality help portray the overall burden of disease in society.[14] This raises methodology concerns, specifically the adding-up constraint: it is not always entirely clear what costs are associated with each disease and how to ensure that all medical spending is allocated to one and only one disease.[14] For analysts using retrospective datasets, the attribution of costs to a particular disease can be difficult, especially if patients have several other medical conditions. Moreover, despite the popularity of COI studies, it is surprising that there is little published guidance to support the choice of methodological approach to be used. Therefore, many COI studies in the United States are not comparable because they differ in terms of the valuation approaches used, the perspective adopted, and the components of care analyzed.[15]

WHAT IS THE REPORTED ECONOMIC BURDEN OF HNC IN THE UNITED STATES?

A literature review was conducted to ascertain the published data regarding the economic burden of HNC. This review builds on previous economic reviews of HNC.[16–18] The initial search strategy was performed in PubMed. Multiple searches using various terms pertaining to costs and the site of disease were used. Supplemental databases searches were also performed (see Appendix for search strategy). As a review, it is a summary of the literature specifically relevant to the United States but more tellingly it critiques the HPV dimension of economic studies on HNC. Seven studies were identified that reported estimates of direct medical costs and productivity losses.

Of these, 2 of the 7 studies (**Table 1**) estimated the economic burden of HPV-associated HNC over a patient's lifetime. Hu and Goldie[19] base their estimates on a previous study by Lang and colleagues[21] that looked at Medicare patients. From the epidemiologic evidence, we know that HPV-associated HNC are predominately in patients aged 40 to 59 years, whereas Medicare claims are based on patients aged older than 65 years. This is the main shortcoming in using this data source. Also, it should be noted that the evaluated patients were from 1991 through 1993, when combined modality therapy had not come into play.[22]

In 2008, a National Cancer Institute (NCI) State of the Science meeting used these studies to estimate the annual cost of HPV-associated oropharyngeal cancers. The cost of treatment and disease management was calculated to be in the order of $151 million.[23] It is likely that this figure is a conservative estimate of the treatment cost burden because the cost of the treatment has increased substantially with multiple modality regimens coupled with the increased incidence of HPV-associated cancers.

An analysis by the Centers for Disease Control and Prevention (CDC) reported on the societal burden of mortality due to HPV-associated cancer sites for 2003.[20] The investigators used a human capital approach to estimate the mortality burden in terms of years of potential life lost and mortality-related productivity costs. Specific to oral

Table 1
Economic burden studies of HPV-associated HNC

Author, Year, and Type of Patients	Cost Methodology	Data Sources	Cost Estimates	Main Conclusion and Limitation	HPV Perspective
Hu & Goldie[19] 2008 Report looked at noncervical HPV-related conditions: oropharyngeal and mouth cancer	Discounted lifetime cost per case expressed in present value. Incidence-based approach applied to costs to estimate economic burden	US-linked SEER-Medicare data (Lang et al 2005). British & Dutch studies used for plausible range. American Cancer Society (2003) incidence rates	Average cost per case of HNC in 2003 is $33,020 (range: [min] $15,340–$46,800 [max])	Total lifetime costs for new cases in 2003: $38.1 million (range: $17.7 million–$54.1 million). Uses SEER-Medicare claims data	Underestimated HPV prevalence (10.7% of all oropharyngeal cancer caused by HPV-16, 18)
Ekwuene et al,[20] 2008 HPV-associated cancers: cancers of the tonsil, tongue, and other oral cavity/pharyngeal cancers	Societal burden of mortality: Mortality, YPLL, value of productivity loss from premature death[a]	SEER. US census. National mortality data: CDC's NCHS National Vital Statistics system. US life tables. ICD-10	Year (2003): Number of deaths: 3379. YPLL: 63,587. YPLL per death = 18.8. PVFLE: $406,061,000	Total mortality costs = $1.37 billion. Productivity loss per death = $406,061. Human capital approach used for productivity loss	Used subsites as proxy for HPV-associated cancers

Abbreviations: CDC, Centers for Disease Control and Prevention; ICD-10, International Classification of Diseases and Related Health Problems 10th Edition; NCHS, National Center for Health Statistics; PVFLE, present value of future lifetime earnings; SEER, Surveillance, Epidemiology and End Results; YPLL, years of potential life lost.

[a] Productivity costs of premature mortality were estimated by multiplying the number of deaths in 2003 (stratified by age, sex, and race/ethnicity) by the present value of future lifetime earnings (PVFLE) stratified by age and sex. The PVFLE estimates that were applied took into account factors like life expectancy, the labor force participation rate and future growth rate in productivity, and the imputed value of housekeeping services (eg, cooking, cleaning, childcare).

cavity/pharynx, they estimated the present future value of lifetime lost productivity of cancer to be $1.37 billion, with men accounting for $1.1.billion.[20] The investigators do not take into account the attributed fraction caused by HPV, which would significantly lower the burden estimate. However, this report does provide an upper bound estimate on what the productivity losses would be if all the cancers were HPV-associated.

WHAT DIRECT MEDICAL COST STUDIES HAVE BEEN CONDUCTED IN THE UNITED STATES?

Five pertinent direct medical cost studies that looked at clinically diverse populations of patients with HNC are given in **Table 2**. The range of patients evaluated, the cost methodology adopted, the length of data collection, and the data sources used differ among the studies. All of these studies used the *International Classification of Diseases, Ninth Revision (ICD-9)* and *Tenth Revision (ICD-10)* codes as the basis of their disease diagnosis. However, none of these studies considered HPV-association with HNC. Perhaps only an ICD code indicating the HPV status of patients with HNC would facilitate an accurate characterization of the economic burden of HPV-associated HNC. It should be noted that Ekwuene and colleagues[20] (see **Table 1**) used cancers of the tonsil, tongue, and "other oral cavity/pharyngeal" cancers as a proxy for HPV-associated HNC. These sites are the specific sites where HPV-associated cancers develop, and it is the cost-of-care estimates associated with these sites that are of particular interest. Fortunately, the Longitudinal Oncology Registry of Head and Neck Carcinoma (LORHAN) are tracking whether HPV testing is being performed.[27] Hopefully, future cost studies may avail of stratification by HPV status.

Two studies (Lang and Epstein[21,26]) used exclusively publicly funded cost sources. Such cost data refer to payments for services paid for by the state/federal government for a subset of the general population. These studies use public payment rates that may underestimate the economic burden of the disease. As noted in a study (Choi and colleagues[25]) using a large US commercial managed care claims database (n = 6570), the average first-year expenditures associated with HNC diagnosis in this population ($29,608 ± 77,500) is higher than the projected average Medicare payment ($18,000). The other two studies also used private-sector health cost data (Amonkar and colleagues[22] and Le and colleagues[24]). They highlight the direct medical costs associated with specific types of patients with HNC: treated with surgery or diagnosed with metastatic or recurrent locally advanced cancer. For purposes of collecting data on HPV-associated HNC, the essential first step is to obtain an accurate, standardized, HPV status so that future analysis can refer to confirmed HPV-positive HNC.

WHAT ARE THE COSTS INVOLVED IN DIAGNOSIS, TREATMENT, AND MANAGEMENT OF HNC?

Various choices exist in how to diagnose, treat, and manage patients with HNC. In the 2011 National Comprehensive Cancer Network (NCCN) guidelines, testing for tumor HPV is suggested and immunohistochemical staining for the surrogate biomarker p16 is recommended.[28] It is likely that HPV/p16 testing will become common practice, but a standardized method has not emerged thus far. A recent survey performed in the United Kingdom reported that the associated laboratory resources (ie, to determine HPV status) cost between £45 and £60. The cost is borne by the publically funded National Health Service (NHS) and depends on the HPV detection technique.[29] In the United States, a more nuanced payment structure for diagnostic services exists. For a general summary of Medicare coverage, coding, and payment for therapeutic and diagnostic devices, refer to Ackerman and colleagues's[30] (2011) edited book: *Therapeutic and Diagnostic Device*

Table 2
The pertinent US cost studies that look at a clinical diverse population of patients with HNC and the HPV perspective

Author, Year, and Type of Patients	Cost Methodology	Data Sources	Cost Estimates	Main Conclusion and Limitation	HPV Perspective
Amonkar et al,[22] 2011 Resected SCCHN (N = 1104)	Retrospective claims-based analysis of commercially insured patients (2004–2007)	Medical, pharmacy, and laboratory data & enrollment information from a large US database of commercially insured patients	Patients incurred ~ $94 million in costs following index surgery (average: $85,000 per patient [2008 USD]). Mean total health care cost was $34,450 per patient per year (2008 USD).	Patients with resected SCCHN incur substantial health care costs and have high use rates Managed care setting, not generalizable	Not mentioned in report ICD-9 codes used to identify patients Possible to separate by HPV-associated subsites
Le et al,[24] 2011 Metastatic (N = 1042) & recurrent, locally advanced (N = 324) HNC	Retrospective payer-based analysis (2004–2008) Compared rate frequency and costs of health care use during the 6 mo after index period	Thomson MarketScan databases (Medicare data & private-sector health data from ~100 payers)	Any-cause total health care costs: • Patients with unadjusted metastatic HNC (n = 1042) = $65,412 ± $74,181 (2008 USD) • Patients with unadjusted recurrent locally advanced HNC (n = 324) = $25,837 ± $43,460 (2008 USD)	"Advanced HNC patients, pose a significant health economic burden on the payer" Based on patients receiving employer-sponsored health insurance, not generalizable	Not mentioned in poster ICD-9 codes used to identify patients Possible to separate by HPV-associated subsites
Choi et al,[25] 2009 HNC diagnosis (N = 6570)	First -year expenditures associated with HNC diagnosis in the US managed care population	US commercial managed care claims database	Projected average Medicare payment per individual in 1 y after HNC diagnosis = $18,000 (2007 USD) Average heath care cost per patient 1 y after HNC diagnosis = $29,608 (±$77,500) (2007 USD)	Annual cost associated with HNC is higher in the managed care population than reported on Medicare population	Not mentioned in abstract ICD-9 codes used to identify patients Possible to separate by HPV-associated subsites

Epstein et al,[26] 2007 OSCC and pharyngeal squamous cell carcinoma (N = 3422)	Direct medical costs of patients were defined as being treated for early or late-stage disease based on treatment modality	Retrospective analysis of California Medicaid claims data CPT-4 coding in claims data	Median year-1 cost of care following initial diagnosis = $25,319 (n = 229) (2002 USD) Estimated range of year-1 cost of care in a commercial PPO in California = $42,198–$72,340 (2002 USD)	Costs for patients treated as having early stage OSCC were approximately 36% less than those treated with late-stage disease (P = .002). Did not include patients that died within 1 y of diagnosis	Not mentioned in report ICD-9 codes used to identify patients Possible to separate by HPV-associated subsites
Lang et al,[21] 2004 Retrospective cohort analysis of newly diagnosed elderly (>65 y) SCCHN (N = 4536)	Linked clinical data to Medicare claims	SEER and Medicare claims Selected diagnosis-related groups, ICD-9-CM diagnosis and procedure codes, and Healthcare Common Procedure Coding System codes in the Medicare claims data	Total mean Medicare payments = $48,847 IQ range: $16,314–$65,682 (1998 USD) Average Medicare payments among patients with SCCHN were $25,542 higher than those of the matched comparison group (P<.001) (1998 USD)	Patients with advanced SCCHN had shorter survival and higher costs than patients diagnosed as having distant, regional, local, and in situ cancer Medicare looks at patients aged >65 y; data 1991–1993	Not mentioned in report ICD-9 codes used to identify patients Possible to separate by HPV-associated subsites

Abbreviations: CPT-4, Current Procedure Terminology codes; *ICD-9, International Classification of Diseases and Related Health Problems 9th Edition;* OSCC, oral squamous cell carcinoma; PPO, preferred provider organization; SCCHN, squamous cell carcinoma of the head and neck; USD, United States dollars.

Outcomes Research. The charge to Medicare is likely to be part of a single bundled payment for the facility's services furnished to a Medicare beneficiary coupled with the physician fees.

It should be noted that the identification of a novel biomarker, such as HPV or p16, would never make economic sense if it were not clinically useful.[31] Currently, the NCCN and others note that the results of HPV testing should not change management decisions except in the context of a clinical trial.[4,28] Historically, HNC, whether or not associated with HPV, have been treated in the same manner.[32] However, it has been suggested from multiple retrospective case series that patients with HPV-positive HNC have an improved overall prognosis.[7,32–36] Moreover, the literature calls for less-intense treatment strategies that do not compromise survival outcomes but lower the risk of debilitating side effects in HPV-positive HNC.[3]

Currently, clinicians and patients are faced with a variety of treatment modalities with huge uncertainties regarding the best sequence of treatment.[37,38] In 2010, the Cochrane Library conducted systematic reviews on the 3 broad treatment modalities in HNC (surgery, radiation, and chemotherapy), although there was little reference to HPV status.[39–41] An optimal treatment algorithm based on HPV and smoking status will likely occur once the results from clinical trials are known.

Treatment: Surgery

A 2007 review identified 6 costing studies on various treatment strategies for HNC of which 5 involved some form of surgery in the treatment algorithm.[16] Since that review, a study using data from the Maryland Health Service Cost Review Commission database identified attributes to the cost of surgery for oropharyngeal cancer surgical cases (1990–2009).[42] These cost drivers were:

- Postoperative wound complications
- Length of hospital stay
- In-hospital death.

For patients aged younger than 60 years (n = 735), the mean cost of hospital care was \$24,537 (median \$19,655; range: minimum \$1493 and maximum \$298,032 in 2009).[42] These figures did not include physician-related costs and that hospital-related charges for each index admission were converted to the organizational cost of providing care using cost-to-charge ratios for individual hospitals.[42]

As noted in a study using case reviews (n = 100) from one US medical facility, post-operative medical complications were statistically far more important in negatively affecting the outcomes and true costs of microsurgical reconstruction for patients with HNC than microsurgical complications.[43] Perhaps the cost of surgery in HNC depends more on the physical condition of patients and not just the progression of the disease. As noted, patients who are HPV positive are generally younger and healthier than patients who are HPV negative.

A promising development in surgery is the use of minimally invasive transoral robotic surgery (TORS) for difficult-to-access cancers. TORS represents the surgical equivalent of delivering targeted therapy for HNC.[44]

Treatment: Radiation Therapy

A nonoperative approach is favored for patients with HNC for whom surgery followed by either radiation therapy (RT) alone or radio chemotherapy may lead to severe functional impairment.[45] In an expert review piece, David Sher[46] highlighted that no cost-effectiveness-analysis (CEA) studies have been performed evaluating the use of radiation therapy for HNC. CEA is a form of full economic evaluation whereby both the costs and consequences of alternative health programs or treatments are examined and compared between treatment options with consequences most often measured in natural units (eg, cost per millimeters of mercury decrease in diastolic blood pressure).[47] In light of the better prognosis of patients with HPV-positive HNC, the focus is to reduce the treatment morbidity. Hence, the Eastern Cooperative Oncology Group and the Radiation Therapy Oncology Group are planning a complex treatment regimen with lower dose radiation (Total dose 54 Gy, conventional dose 70 Gy).[3]

For advanced cancers, the RT is usually delivered with more expensive intensity-modulated RT (IMRT) and there is also interest in using proton beam therapy (PBT).[48] The increase in the use of IMRT and PBT is expected to further add to national expenditures on RT services.[46] Again, Sher states that there is a clear need for a CEA comparing IMRT and PBT with 3-dimensional conformal RT in head and neck squamous cell carcinomas.[46]

Treatment: Chemotherapy

Chemotherapy is often used in combination with RT for treating patients with HNC. In a recent review (2011), chemotherapy in HNC includes one or a combination of the following: cisplatin, carboplatin, 5-fluorouracil, paclitaxel, docetaxel, leucovorin, and cetuximab.[37] In a managed-care population (2004–2007), the mean 2008 US dollar figure for total chemotherapy cost per patient per year was $2004 for pharyngeal cancer (n = 185) and $1177 for lip/tongue cancer (n = 367). This cost is considerably less than the total mean radiation cost of $11,833 and $7264 for pharyngeal and lip/tongue cancer respectively.[22]

The LORHAN group reported that for 1144 patients, inexpensive (~$40/100 mg vial) cisplatin-based chemotherapy was the most frequently used regimen (51%) and that the vastly more expensive ($10,000+ per treatment cycle) cetuximab was the next most commonly used regimen (21%) in the United States.[27] One of the secondary aims of Clinical trial NCT01302834 is to explore differences in the cost-effectiveness of cetuximab as compared with cisplatin in HPV-associated oropharynx cancer. Cetuximab, a monoclonal antibody inhibitor, works by antagonizing the epidermal growth factor receptor (EGFR). HPV and p16 status is important to determine the prognostic value; however, EGFR status has a predictive treatment value. An Australian study showed that only 2 of 126 patients (1.6%) with oropharyngeal cancer were found to be p16+/EGFR fluorescence in situ hybridization positive.[49] This finding may suggest that cetuximab may not be appropriate for all HPV-associated HNC.

Cost of Posttreatment Management

One of the significant features about all 3 modalities is the risk of complications associated with each treatment option. From an economic perspective, other direct medical costs related to rehabilitation with auxiliary health care professionals and the cost of treatment complications ought to be factored into any cost analysis. Using a retrospective cohort study (PharMetrics Patient-Centric Database 2000–2006), Lang and colleagues[50] found significantly higher rates of treatment-related complications among patients receiving chemoradiotherapy (86%) than among patients receiving radiotherapy alone (51%) ($P<.001$). The mean per-patient costs associated with treatment-related complications were approximately $10,000 higher among patients who received chemoradiotherapy than those treated with radiotherapy alone ($P<.001$).[50] These costs represented 17% of the total costs during follow-up for patients who received chemoradiotherapy and 11% of costs for those who received radiotherapy.

Other US studies have also examined the cost of radiation-induced oral mucositis[51,52] on managing dysphagia[53] and xerostomia[54] in patients with HNC. Treatment options have an array of severe acute toxicities and long-term morbidities that have not been fully documented and are particularly concerning in younger patients with highly curable HPV-associated oropharyngeal cancers.[4] Therefore, it is likely that treatment-related morbidities impose substantial unnecessary costs on patients and payers.

WHAT ARE THE LONG-TERM CARE IMPLICATIONS?

A meta-analysis of 37 studies suggested that patients with HPV-associated HNC had a lower risk of recurrence (meta hazard ratio: 0.62; 95% confidence interval: 0.5–0.8) as compared with HNC patients not associated with HPV.[55] Second primary malignancy (SPM) represents the leading long-term cause of mortality in patients with HNC.[56] Using the Surveillance, Epidemiology, and End Results (SEER) population-based cohort study (n = 75,087 patients with head and neck squamous cell carcinoma), it was found in a trends analysis study that during the HPV era, SPM risk associated with oropharyngeal cancer has declined to the lowest risk level of any head and neck subsites.[57]

Other US studies highlight some of the pertinent issues related to the optimization of surveillance strategies[58] and the supportive-care costs of HNC.[59] Follow-up strategies of HPV-associated HNC have obvious cost implications; as the results of clinical trials mature, the optimal strategy for the surveillance of patients with HPV-associated HNC will also emerge. The direct medical costs along the care continuum for patients with HPV-associated HNC is not a trivial issue. Hence, a budget impact analysis (BIA) model would be a useful tool for health care providers who manage these patients. BIA should be performed using data that reflect, for a specific health condition, the size and characteristics of the population, the current and new treatment mix, the efficacy and safety of the new and current treatments, and the resource use and costs for the treatments and symptoms that would apply to the population of interest.[60]

WHAT ARE THE PRODUCTIVITY LOSSES AND INTANGIBLE COSTS?

Treatment-related productivity losses (indirect costs) incurred by sick-leave days taken to treat and recover from an HPV-associated HNC are likely to be substantial. A French study estimated the mean number of workdays lost (absenteeism) to be 120; in calculating the cost of productivity losses, they assigned a monetary compensation or daily allowance that is given by the health care payer to partially offset the patients' loss of income.[61] A German study estimates that sick leave accounts for 16% of the total costs in their HPV-associated HNC COI study.[62] Furthermore, there is also the controversial issue of including presenteeism, (the effect of poor health on job productivity) in COI studies. Unfortunately, an estimate of the prevalence costs associated with sick leave/productivity losses has not been calculated in the United States. Ekwueme and colleagues[20] calculated the incident costs (the lifetime lost productivity of those who died of cancer in 2003).

Intangible costs are defined as the pain and suffering of patients because of a disease, which are usually measured by the reduction in quality of life. Recent examples in the literature relate to arthritis.[63,64] One method of estimating the monetary value of intangible costs is the contingent valuation method, a stated preference method based on the elicitation of levels of willingness to pay; an example is valuing a hypothetical cure for rheumatoid arthritis.[65] It remains controversial to value intangible costs in monetary terms because no real market exists and it is often overlooked in COI studies.[63]

COI OF HPV-ASSOCIATED HNC IN THE UNITED STATES: WHAT HAS AND HAS NOT BEEN ESTIMATED?

The NCI reported that in 2006 approximately $3.1 billion was spent in the United States each year on HNC treatment, which is the 10th most expensive cancer to treat.[66] The CDC estimated the average number of incident cases per year between 2003 and 2007 to be 10,752 in potential HPV-associated sites.[67] This figure is about 30% of the estimated new cancer cases of all oral cavity and pharynx cancers (n = 36,540) in the United States in 2010.[68] The figure of the annual cost of HPV-associated HNC can be crudely estimated from the proportion that is then attributable to HPV, possibly around $650 million (If the total HNC treatment cost is $3.1 billion, then 30% of these are HPV-associated HNC sites and ~70–80% of cancers in these sites are HPV positive).

An attempt to summarize the COI components of HPV-associated HNC in the United States has been described in **Table 3**. The table contains the pertinent estimates that have been extracted from the literature that describe the economic burden by what is termed the societal perspective. This perspective is what is recommended for CEA in the United States.[70] Many outstanding methodology issues remain in using this perspective.[71] A narrower perspective is that of the third-party payer, the health insurer or government agency. Often the payer is only interested in the direct medical costs of patients that are borne by them. The purpose of describing the economic burden/COI is to highlight to policy makers the savings that can be made if this illness were eradicated.

WHAT ARE THE CHALLENGES FACING THE USE OF ECONOMIC DATA IN HPV-ASSOCIATED HNC IN THE UNITED STATES?

There are several challenges facing the use of economic data for HPV-associated HNC in the United States. Without ICD codes indicating to an analyst that a patient has HPV-positive HNC, the default approach will be reference to HPV-associated HNC sites adjusted by the percentage that are HPV positive from other studies. Subsequently, US cost databases (eg, Medicare claims, hospital administrative, and so forth) will not be truly accurate in characterizing the economic burden of this new disease entity.

On a health care system level, many health technology assessment agencies around the globe use the quality-adjusted life-year (QALY), which is a generic outcome measure used in CEA and cost-utility analysis (CUA). The QALY is a measure of disease burden, including both the quality and quantity of life lived. CUA is a form of evaluation that focuses particular attention on the quality of the health outcome produced or foregone by health programs or treatments. Outcomes in CUA are generic rather than program specific and incorporate the notion of value (eg, cost per QALY gained).[47] In the United States, spending $50,000 to improve health by one QALY has been discussed as a threshold to determine whether a technology is cost-effective.[72] However, there is no clear evidence that the Centers for Medicare and Medicaid Services uses such an implicit threshold in the decision-making process for their National Coverage Decisions.[73] As part of the Patient Protection and Affordable Care Act, the QALY or other such generic health measures cannot be used in the decision-making process of federal agencies.[74]

Table 3
Characterizing the COI of HPV-associated HNC

Components to Characterize the COI	Authors	Notes
Direct medical costs	NCI Report[67]	*All HNC:* $3.1billion per year (2006 USD) • Initial care ($0.9 billion; 29.5%): the first 12 mo after diagnosis • Continuing care ($0.8 billion; 28.1%): time between initial and last year of life • Last year of life ($1.3 billion; 42.4%): the final 12 mo of life
	Chaturvedi[23]	*HPV-associated oropharyngeal cancer:* $151 million per year (2003 USD)
Cost per case	Hu and Goldie[19]	*Oropharyngeal and mouth cancer:* $33,020 (2003 USD) is the average discounted lifetime cost per case. *HPV-associated oropharyngeal and mouth cancer:* Total discounted lifetime cost for HNC in 2003 is $38.1 million (range: $17.7–$54.1 million).
Indirect medical costs	n/a	No estimate of these costs has been reported
Productivity losses	Bradley et al[69]	*All HNC:* $3.6 billion – PVLE among adults aged ≧20 y in 2010 USD based on 12,109 deaths; PVLE/death = $299,809
	Ekwuene et al[20]	*HPV-associated HNC sites:* $1.37 billion (2003 USD)
Intangible costs	n/a	No estimate of these costs has been reported

Abbreviations: n/a, not available; PVLE, present value of lifetime earnings; USD, United States dollars.

In medical research, it is not uncommon to conduct economic evaluations alongside clinical trials, although these economic studies suffer the same external validity issues that accompany any finding from a randomized trial. Therefore, it would be prudent to enlist an experienced health economist at the earliest stage possible into the trial design team. Establishing the appropriate time frame for the evaluation of patients' complications is crucial to an accurate economic evaluation of patients with HNC.[75]

WHAT CONTROVERSIES ARE ASSOCIATED WITH USING ECONOMIC DATA?

The overarching controversies surrounding HPV-associated HNC relate to the implications for prevention.[3,76–78] Potentially, the 2 main prevention methods are by

Oral cancer screening
HPV prophylactic vaccination

Recently, a Markov decision analysis approach was used to assess the cost-effectiveness of community-based screening for oral cancer in the United States.[79] Unfortunately, it is unlikely that any current visual/cytologic evaluation screening method will detect HPV-associated oropharyngeal cancer because of its difficult-to-examine anatomic position.[80] Fakhry and colleagues[81] have shown that the cytologic evaluation of the oropharynx, although useful in detecting invasive oropharyngeal cancers, may have limited utility as a screening modality for detecting precancerous cells.[81,82] The issue of beneficial population-level screening relates to effectiveness and not cost-effectiveness.

Whether giving HPV prophylactic vaccination to boys and girls is cost-effective is a topic of much debate.[83,84] If HPV vaccination prevents all noncervical HPV-positive cancers, this would substantially increase its cost-effectiveness.[85] A meta-analysis that looked at the impact of HPV on cancer risk in HNC reported that, in the context of their findings, "it is conceivable that extending vaccination to both sexes would prevent a significant number of future oropharyngeal cancers in both men and women."[86] In October 2011, the CDC's Advisory Committee on Immunization Practices recommended that the HPV vaccine series be given to boys aged 11 to 12 years, and as an independent expert advisory board, they can consider CEA in their deliberations.[87]

WHAT FUTURE ECONOMIC RESEARCH INTO HPV-HNC WOULD BE BENEFICIAL?

Research into establishing the most effective and cost-effective HPV detection method in HNC would be a timely addition to the literature. As a CEA, the outcome would put a dollar amount on the cost per case of HPV-positive HNC detected. Investigation in the optimal treatment paradigm of HPV-positive HNC depends on the results of numerous clinical trials (eg, NCT01084083, NCT01302834, NCT01111942). Thus far, no cost-effectiveness studies have been performed evaluating the use of the different modalities for HNC.

In the spirit of characterizing HPV-associated HNC as a separate disease entity, a cost study comparing the resource use of newly diagnosed patients who are HPV positive and HPV negative from the same anatomic site (controlling for smoking status and other covariates) would also be informative to health care managers and researchers. Such a study would give an accurate cost per case of a patient who is HPV positive. The importance of an accurate cost-per-case estimate is that these figures are used as the input values in economic models that evaluate interventions, such as the HPV vaccine.[88]

A French study that used their National Hospital Database to estimate the total costs associated with HPV-associated cancers in France illustrates the substantial burden of HPV-associated HNC. The total costs for all HPV-associated cancer in both sexes were estimated to be €239.7 million (US $346.4 million). The overall costs in men were €107.2 million (US $154.9 million), driven mainly by HNC (€94.6 million, US $136.7 million).[61] In the United States, the Medical Expenditure Panel Survey (MEPS) has been used as a data source to characterize the costs of other conditions[89,90] and to estimate associated productivity losses.[91,92] MEPS data should help characterize the direct medical expenditures of HNC but not HPV-associated HNC. For national hospital statistics, the Healthcare Cost and Utilization Project (HCUP) is also available. Both MEPS and HCUP are maintained by the US Agency for Healthcare Research and Quality.

SUMMARY

A major improvement in characterizing the economic impact of HPV-associated HNC in the United States would be the recognition that the cancer is different from traditional HNC. The annual direct medical costs are likely to be more than the 2008 estimate of $151 million but a lot less than the NCI's 2006 figure of $3.1 billion for all HNC. Although there are more diagnosed cases of HPV-positive HNC now, the trend is to treat these cases less intensively than patients with traditional HNC. The net cost or savings of medical costs would be extremely difficult to determine given current data sources. However, there is likely to be a substantial burden implied by the productivity losses and intangible costs suffered by patients who are overtreated in the absence of a straightforward diagnostic test.

Should clinicians or patients care about these economic studies? As noted in an editorial referring to a study on productivity losses caused by cancer:[69] "perhaps the primary benefit of monetary estimates is simply to translate what professionals and patients already know about the human costs of cancer into a metric that is universally understood. As a tool for advocacy, dollar values can be powerful, particularly when they are weighed against other programs that influence human life and health under limited budgets."[93]

APPENDIX: LITERATURE REVIEW SEARCH STRATEGY

The inclusion criteria were that the report addressed the costs of HNC in the United States; patients were aged older than 18 years; the study was published in English; and the study was published between 2000 and November 2011. Exclusion criteria included non-US studies, no dollar amounts reported, and we excluded studies that concentrated on HNC subsites not associated with HPV.

The initial search strategy was performed in PubMed. Searches of the following supplemental resources were then performed: Embase, Cochrane Library, Scopus, Web of Science, Medline, Cancerlit, the SEER program (from the National Cancer Institute online database), and the American Society of Clinical Oncology (ASCO) proceedings (2000–2011). The economic databases searched included the following: Econlit, the Cost-Effectiveness Analysis (CEA) registry, Center for Reviews and Dissemination (CRD), NHS Economic Evaluation Database (EED), the International Society for Pharmacoeconomics and Outcomes Research (ISPOR) proceedings (2000–2011), and the Society for Medical Decision Making (SMDM) proceedings (2000–2011). Other sources included www.clinicaltrials.gov and the International Standard Randomized Controlled Trial Number (ISRCTN) registry. Comprehensive Internet searches using well-known search engines (eg, Google Scholar) were also conducted to assist in the search for published articles.

To begin the search, the following broad Medical Subject Headings (MeSH) and text-only search terms were used: "Head and neck neoplasms" (MeSH) AND "Economics" (MeSH) restricted to the English language, aged 19 years and older, and a publication date between 2000 and 2012. The initial search generated 253 references in PubMed. Other searches included combining key words, such as cost and cost analysis with human papillomavirus, oropharyngeal cancer, oral cancer, mouth cancer, and head and neck cancer. Abstracts were reviewed from each reference and any references thought to be relevant were retrieved in full text. Specifically, studies were retrieved in full text if they contained any cost information regarding the economic burden associated with the screening, diagnosis, or treatment of HPV-associated HNC. The electronic search was supplemented by a manual review of the bibliographies of review articles and original research articles that had been retrieved. We screened all full-text articles for final inclusion in the analysis and found 7 articles to be included of which 2 were abstracts from ISPOR conferences.

The objective is to identify HNC costing studies reported in the United States. Outcomes of interest are associated cost-of-treatment estimates. Only original study design (reviews and hypothetical models excluded) with defined populations and economic end points were considered. Those publications that met these criteria were then reviewed carefully, and a systematic evaluation was made of the pertinent characteristics of the study (sample size, population), the cost analysis, and the findings. The costs provided in the article are the original data reported in the studies.

REFERENCES

1. Sturgis EM, Cinciripini PM. Trends in head and neck cancer incidence in relation to smoking prevalence: an emerging epidemic of human papillomavirus-associated cancers? Cancer 2007;110(7):1429–35.
2. Näsman A, Attner P, Hammarstedt L, et al. Incidence of human papillomavirus (HPV) positive tonsillar carcinoma in Stockholm, Sweden: an epidemic of viral-induced carcinoma? Int J Cancer 2009;125(2):362–6.
3. Marur S, D'Souza G, Westra WH, et al. HPV-associated head and neck cancer: a virus-related cancer epidemic. Lancet Oncol 2010;11(8):781–9.
4. Sturgis EM, Ang KK. The epidemic of HPV-associated oropharyngeal cancer is here: is it time to change our treatment paradigms? J Natl Compr Canc Netw 2011;9(6):665–73.
5. Chaturvedi AK, Engels EA, Pfeiffer RM, et al. Human papillomavirus and rising oropharyngeal cancer incidence in the United States. J Clin Oncol 2011; 29(32):4294–301.
6. D'Souza G, Agrawal Y, Halpern J, et al. Oral sexual behaviors associated with prevalent oral human papillomavirus infection. J Infect Dis 2009;199(9):1263–9.
7. Adelstein DJ, Rodriguez CP. Human papillomavirus: changing paradigms in oropharyngeal cancer. Curr Oncol Rep 2010;12(2):115–20.
8. Gillison ML. Human papillomavirus-associated head and neck cancer is a distinct epidemiologic, clinical, and molecular entity. Semin Oncol 2004;31(6):744–54.
9. Kreimer AR. Oral sexual behaviors and the prevalence of oral human papilloma-virus infection. J Infect Dis 2009;199(9):1253–4.
10. Landro L. Throat cancer linked to virus [Internet]. wsjcom. 2011. Available at: http://online.wsj.com/article/SB10001424052702303657404576355403363380510.html. Accessed June 11, 2012.
11. Frick KD, Kymes SM. The calculation and use of economic burden data. Br J Ophthalmol 2006;90(3):255–7.
12. van Monsjou HS, Balm AJM, van den Brekel MM, et al. Oropharyngeal squamous cell carcinoma: a unique disease on the rise? Oral Oncol 2010;46(11):780–5.
13. Larg A, Moss JR. Cost-of-illness studies: a guide to critical evaluation. Pharma-coeconomics 2011;29(8):653–71.
14. Rosen AB, Cutler DM. Challenges in building disease-based national health accounts. Med Care 2009;47(7 Suppl 1):S7–13.
15. Clabaugh G, Ward MM. Cost-of-illness studies in the United States: a systematic review of methodologies used for direct cost. Value Health 2008;11(1):13–21.
16. Menzin J, Lines LM, Manning LN. The economics of squamous cell carcinoma of the head and neck. Curr Opin Otolaryngol Head Neck Surg 2007;15(2): 68–73.
17. Lee JM, Turini M, Botteman MF, et al. Economic burden of head and neck cancer. A literature review. Eur J Health Econ 2004;5(1):70–80.
18. Selke B, Allenet B, Bercez C, et al. Economic assessments of head and neck cancers: a review. Bull Cancer 2001;88(8):759–64.
19. Hu D, Goldie S. The economic burden of noncervical human papillomavirus disease in the United States. Am J Obstet Gynecol 2008;198(5):500 e1–7.

20. Ekwueme DU, Chesson HW, Zhang KB, et al. Years of potential life lost and productivity costs because of cancer mortality and for specific cancer sites where human papillomavirus may be a risk factor for carcinogenesis-United States, 2003. Cancer 2008;113(Suppl 10):2936–45.

21. Lang K, Menzin J, Earle CC, et al. The economic cost of squamous cell cancer of the head and neck: findings from linked SEER-Medicare data. Arch Otolaryngol Head Neck Surg 2004;130(11):1269–75.

22. Amonkar MM, Chastek B, Samant N, et al. Economic burden of resected squamous cell carcinoma of the head and neck in a US managed-care population. J Med Econ 2011;14(4):421–32.

23. Adelstein DJ, Ridge JA, Gillison ML, et al. Head and neck squamous cell cancer and the human papillomavirus: summary of a National Cancer Institute State of the Science Meeting, November 9-10, 2008, Washington, D.C. Head Neck 2009;31(11):1393–422.

24. Le TK, Winfree KB, Yang H, et al. Health care resource utilization and economic burden of metastatic and recurrent locally-advanced head and neck cancer patients. Value Health 2011;14(3):A172–3.

25. Choi J, Joish V, Camacho F, et al. First year cost expenditures associated with head and neck cancer diagnosis in the U.S. managed care population. Value Health 2009;12(3):A47–8.

26. Epstein JD, Knight TK, Epstein JB, et al. Cost of care for early- and late-stage oral and pharyngeal cancer in the California Medicaid population. Head Neck 2008; 30(2):178–86.

27. Wong SJ, Harari PM, Garden AS, et al. Longitudinal Oncology Registry of Head and Neck Carcinoma (LORHAN): analysis of chemoradiation treatment approaches in the United States. Cancer 2011;117(8):1679–86.

28. NCCN clinical practice guidelines in oncology [Internet]. Available at: http://www.nccn.org/professionals/physician_gls/f_guidelines.asp. Accessed July 22, 2011.

29. Ahmed A, Cascarini L, Sandison A, et al. Survey of the use of tests for human papilloma virus and epidermal growth factor receptor for squamous cell carcinoma of the head and neck in UK head and neck multidisciplinary teams [Internet]. Br J Oral Maxillofac Surg 2011;50(2):119–21.

30. Ackerman SJ, Smith MD, Ehreth J, et al. Therapeutic and diagnostic device outcomes research. Lawrenceville (NJ): ISPOR; 2011.

31. Scott MG. When do new biomarkers make economic sense? Scand J Clin Lab Invest Suppl 2010;242:90–5.

32. Sedaghat AR, Zhang Z, Begum S, et al. Prognostic significance of human papillomavirus in oropharyngeal squamous cell carcinomas. Laryngoscope 2009; 119(8):1542–9.

33. Fakhry C, Westra WH, Li S, et al. Improved survival of patients with human papillomavirus-positive head and neck squamous cell carcinoma in a prospective clinical trial. J Natl Cancer Inst 2008;100(4):261–9.

34. Weinberger PM, Yu Z, Haffty BG, et al. Molecular classification identifies a subset of human papillomavirus–associated oropharyngeal cancers with favorable prognosis. J Clin Oncol 2006;24(5):736–47.

35. Licitra L, Perrone F, Bossi P, et al. High-risk human papillomavirus affects prognosis in patients with surgically treated oropharyngeal squamous cell carcinoma. J Clin Oncol 2006;24(36):5630–6.

36. Reimers N, Kasper HU, Weissenborn SJ, et al. Combined analysis of HPV-DNA, p16 and EGFR expression to predict prognosis in oropharyngeal cancer. Int J Cancer 2007;120(8):1731–8.

37. Tribius S, Ihloff AS, Rieckmann T, et al. Impact of HPV status on treatment of squamous cell cancer of the oropharynx: what we know and what we need to know. Cancer Lett 2011;304(2):71–9.
38. Ihloff AS, Petersen C, Hoffmann M, et al. Human papilloma virus in locally advanced stage III/IV squamous cell cancer of the oropharynx and impact on choice of therapy. Oral Oncol 2010;46(10):705–11.
39. Oliver RJ, Clarkson JE, Conway DI, et al. Interventions for the treatment of oral and oropharyngeal cancers: surgical treatment. Cochrane Database Syst Rev 2007;4:CD006205.
40. Furness S, Glenny AM, Worthington HV, et al. Interventions for the treatment of oral cavity and oropharyngeal cancer: chemotherapy. Cochrane Database Syst Rev 2011;4:CD006386.
41. Glenny AM, Furness S, Worthington HV, et al. Interventions for the treatment of oral cavity and oropharyngeal cancer: radiotherapy. Cochrane Database Syst Rev 2010;12:CD006387.
42. Gourin CG, Forastiere AA, Sanguineti G, et al. Impact of surgeon and hospital volume on short-term outcomes and cost of oropharyngeal cancer surgical care. Laryngoscope 2011;121(4):746–52.
43. Jones NF, Jarrahy R, Song JI, et al. Postoperative medical complications–not microsurgical complications–negatively influence the morbidity, mortality, and true costs after microsurgical reconstruction for head and neck cancer. Plast Reconstr Surg 2007;119(7):2053–60.
44. Garden AS, Kies MS, Weber RS. To TORS or not to TORS: but is that the question?: comment on "transoral robotic surgery for advanced oropharyngeal carcinoma". Arch Otolaryngol Head Neck Surg 2010;136(11):1085–7.
45. Goon PK, Stanley MA, Ebmeyer J, et al. HPV & head and neck cancer: a descriptive update. Head Neck Oncol 2009;1:36.
46. Sher DJ. Cost–effectiveness studies in radiation therapy. Expert Rev Pharmacoecon Outcomes Res 2010;10(5):567–82.
47. Drummond M, Sculpher M, Torrance G, et al. Methods for the economic evaluation of health care programmes. 3rd edition. Oxford (United Kingdom): Oxford University Press; 2005.
48. Corvò R. Evidence-based radiation oncology in head and neck squamous cell carcinoma. Radiother Oncol 2007;85(1):156–70.
49. Young RJ, Rischin D, Fisher R, et al. Relationship between epidermal growth factor receptor status, p16(INK4A), and outcome in head and neck squamous cell carcinoma. Cancer Epidemiol Biomarkers Prev 2011;20(6):1230–7.
50. Lang K, Sussman M, Friedman M, et al. Incidence and costs of treatment-related complications among patients with advanced squamous cell carcinoma of the head and neck. Arch Otolaryngol Head Neck Surg 2009;135(6):582–8.
51. Elting LS, Cooksley CD, Chambers MS, et al. Risk, outcomes, and costs of radiation-induced oral mucositis among patients with head-and-neck malignancies. Int J Radiat Oncol Biol Phys 2007;68(4):1110–20.
52. Peterman A, Cella D, Glandon G, et al. Mucositis in head and neck cancer: economic and quality-of-life outcomes. J Natl Cancer Inst Monographs 2001;29:45–51.
53. Aviv JE, Sataloff RT, Cohen M, et al. Cost-effectiveness of two types of dysphagia care in head and neck cancer: a preliminary report. Ear Nose Throat J 2001; 80(8):553–6, 558.
54. Chambers MS, Garden AS, Kies MS, et al. Radiation-induced xerostomia in patients with head and neck cancer: pathogenesis, impact on quality of life, and management. Head Neck 2004;26(9):796–807.

55. Ragin CC, Taioli E. Survival of squamous cell carcinoma of the head and neck in relation to human papillomavirus infection: review and meta-analysis. Int J Cancer 2007;121(8):1813–20.

56. Vikram B. Changing patterns of failure in advanced head and neck cancer. Arch Otolaryngol 1984;110(9):564–5.

57. Morris LG, Sikora AG, Patel SG, et al. Second primary cancers after an index head and neck cancer: subsite-specific trends in the era of human papillomavirus-associated oropharyngeal cancer. J Clin Oncol 2011;29(6):739–46.

58. Kazi R, Manikanthan K, Pathak KA, et al. Head and neck squamous cell cancers: need for an organised time-bound surveillance plan. Eur Arch Otorhinolaryngol 2010;267(12):1969–71.

59. Nonzee NJ, Dandade NA, Patel U, et al. Evaluating the supportive care costs of severe radiochemotherapy-induced mucositis and pharyngitis : results from a Northwestern University Costs of Cancer Program pilot study with head and neck and nonsmall cell lung cancer patients who received care at a county hospital, a Veterans Administration hospital, or a comprehensive cancer care center. Cancer 2008;113(6):1446–52.

60. Mauskopf JA, Sullivan SD, Annemans L, et al. Principles of good practice for budget impact analysis: report of the ISPOR task force on good research prac-tices—budget impact analysis. Value Health 2007;10(5):336–47.

61. Borget I, Abramowitz L, Mathevet P. Economic burden of HPV-related cancers in France. Vaccine 2011;29(32):5245–9.

62. Remy V, Heitland W, Klussmann J, et al. Economic burden of HPV-related head & neck cancer and anal cancers in Germany. Presentation at ISPOR 14th Annual European Congress, Madrid (Spain). November 5–8, 2011.

63. Xie F, Thumboo J, Fong KY, et al. A study on indirect and intangible costs for patients with knee osteoarthritis in Singapore. Value Health 2008;11(Suppl 1):S84–90.

64. Leardini G, Salaffi F, Montanelli R, et al. A multicenter cost-of-illness study on rheumatoid arthritis in Italy. Clin Exp Rheumatol 2002;20(4):505–15.

65. Fautrel B, Clarke AE, Guillemin F, et al. Valuing a hypothetical cure for rheumatoid arthritis using the contingent valuation methodology: the patient perspective. J Rheumatol 2005;32(3):443–53.

66. Cancer trends progress report - costs of cancer care [Internet]. Available at: http://progressreport.cancer.gov/doc_detail.asp?pid=1&did=2009&chid=95&coid=926&mid=. Accessed December 7, 2011.

67. CDC - number of HPV-associated cancer cases per year [Internet]. Available at: http://www.cdc.gov.ezproxy.welch.jhmi.edu/cancer/hpv/statistics/cases.htm. Ac-cessed December 8, 2011.

68. Jemal A, Siegel R, Xu J, et al. Cancer statistics, 2010. CA Cancer J Clin 2010; 60(5):277–300.

69. Bradley CJ, Yabroff KR, Dahman B, et al. Productivity costs of cancer mortality in the United States: 2000-2020. J Natl Cancer Inst 2008;100(24):1763–70.

70. Siegel JE, Weinstein MC, Russell LB, et al. Recommendations for reporting cost-effectiveness analyses. Panel on cost-effectiveness in health and medicine. JAMA 1996;276(16):1339–41.

71. Garrison LP Jr, Mansley EC, Abbott TA 3rd, et al. Good research practices for measuring drug costs in cost-effectiveness analyses: a societal perspective: the ISPOR Drug Cost Task Force report–part II. Value Health 2010;13(1):8–13.

72. Bridges JFP, Onukwugha E, Mullins CD. Healthcare rationing by proxy: cost-effectiveness analysis and the misuse of the $50,000 threshold in the US. Phar-macoeconomics 2010;28(3):175–84.

73. Chambers JD, Neumann PJ, Buxton MJ. Does Medicare have an implicit cost-effectiveness threshold? Med Decis Making 2010;30(4):E14–27.
74. Neumann PJ, Weinstein MC. Legislating against use of cost-effectiveness information. N Engl J Med 2010;363(16):1495–7.
75. Nijdam W, Levendag P, Noever I, et al. Cancer in the oropharynx: cost calculation of different treatment modalities for controlled primaries, relapses and grade III/IV complications. Radiother Oncol 2005;77(1):65–72.
76. Psyrri A, Cohen E. Oropharyngeal cancer: clinical implications of the HPV connection. Ann Oncol 2011;22(5):997–9.
77. D'Souza G, Kreimer AR, Viscidi R, et al. Case-control study of human papillomavirus and oropharyngeal cancer. N Engl J Med 2007;356(19):1944–56.
78. Lowy DR, Munger K. Prognostic implications of HPV in oropharyngeal cancer. N Engl J Med 2010;363(1):82–4.
79. Dedhia RC, Smith KJ, Johnson JT, et al. The cost-effectiveness of community-based screening for oral cancer in high-risk males in the United States: a Markov decision analysis approach. Laryngoscope 2011;121(5):952–60.
80. Lingen MW. Brush-based cytology screening in the tonsils and cervix: there is a difference! Cancer Prev Res (Phila) 2011;4(9):1350–2.
81. Fakhry C, Rosenthal BT, Clark DP, et al. Associations between oral HPV16 infection and cytopathology: evaluation of an oropharyngeal "pap-test equivalent" in high-risk populations. Cancer Prev Res (Phila) 2011;4(9):1378–84.
82. Kreimer AR, Chaturvedi AK. HPV-associated oropharyngeal cancers—are they preventable? Cancer Prev Res (Phila) 2011;4(9):1346–9.
83. Beutels P, Jit M. A brief history of economic evaluation for human papillomavirus vaccination policy. Sex Health 2010;7(3):352–8.
84. Kim JJ. Targeted human papillomavirus vaccination of men who have sex with men in the USA: a cost-effectiveness modelling analysis. Lancet Infect Dis 2010;10(12):845–52.
85. de Kok IM, Habbema JD, van Rosmalen J, et al. Would the effect of HPV vaccination on non-cervical HPV-positive cancers make the difference for its cost-effectiveness? Eur J Cancer 2011;47(3):428–35.
86. Dayyani F, Etzel CJ, Liu M, et al. Meta-analysis of the impact of human papillomavirus (HPV) on cancer risk and overall survival in head and neck squamous cell carcinomas (HNSCC). Head Neck Oncol 2010;2:15.
87. Kim JJ. The role of cost-effectiveness in U.S. vaccination policy. N Engl J Med 2011;365(19):1760–1.
88. Kim JJ, Goldie SJ. Health and economic implications of HPV vaccination in the United States. N Engl J Med 2008;359(8):821–32.
89. Finkelstein EA, Fiebelkorn IC, Wang G. National medical spending attributable to overweight and obesity: how much, and who's paying? Health Aff (Millwood) 2003;(Suppl Web Exclusives). W3-219–W3-226.
90. Hogan P, Dall T, Nikolov P. Economic costs of diabetes in the US in 2002. Diabetes Care 2003;26(3):917–32.
91. Sullivan PW, Ghushchyan VH, Slejko JF, et al. The burden of adult asthma in the United States: evidence from the Medical Expenditure Panel survey. J Allergy Clin Immunol 2011;127(2):363–9, e1–3.
92. Blanciforti LA. Economic burden of dermatitis in US workers [corrected]. J Occup Environ Med 2010;52(11):1045–54.
93. Ramsey SD. How should we value lives lost to cancer? J Natl Cancer Inst 2008;100(24):1742–3.

Index

Note: Page numbers of article titles are in **boldface** type.

Otolaryngol Clin N Am 45 (2012) 919–924
http://dx.doi.org/10.1016/S0030-6665(12)00077-1
0030-6665/12/$ – see front matter © 2012 Elsevier Inc. All rights reserved.

oto.theclinics.com

Moving?

Make sure your subscription moves with you!

To notify us of your new address, find your **Clinics Account Number** (located on your mailing label above your name), and contact customer service at:

Email: journalscustomerservice-usa@elsevier.com

800-654-2452 (subscribers in the U.S. & Canada)
314-447-8871 (subscribers outside of the U.S. & Canada)

Fax number: 314-447-8029

Elsevier Health Sciences Division
Subscription Customer Service
3251 Riverport Lane
Maryland Heights, MO 63043

*To ensure uninterrupted delivery of your subscription, please notify us at least 4 weeks in advance of move.

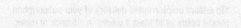